Periodontal Control

Periodontal Control

An Effective System for Diagnosis,
Selection, Control and Treatment
Planning in General Practice

A.M. Grace, BDS
and
F.C. Smales, PhD, BDS, FDS

1989
Quintessence Publishing Co Ltd
London, Chicago, Berlin, Sao Paulo, Tokyo

First published 1989 by
Quintessence Publishing Company Ltd
London, UK

British Library Cataloguing in Publication Data
Grace, A.M.
  Periodontal control
  1. Man. Periodontal diseases
  I. Title II. Smales F.C.
  617.6'32

  ISBN 1-85097-009-2

Printed in Great Britain by Biddles Ltd, Guildford, Surrey, UK
from typesetting by Alacrity Phototypesetters,
Banwell Castle, Weston-super-Mare

Contents

Foreword

by Professor R. Duckworth

*Head of the Department of Oral
Medicine and Periodontology
London Hospital Medical College*

It is remarkable that each of the recent decades have provided a single predominant theme for dentistry. The sixties were notable for a world-wide expansion in the size and complexity of dental education. In the seventies there was a flowering of research in all aspects of dentistry but, above all else, into prevention. The dental theme of the eighties is clearly apparent, as we approach the end of the decade. It is the profound change which has begun to occur in the general dental practice situation as it is being freed from the pandemic of dental caries, only to be assailed simultaneously by a host of social and technological changes.

The contents of this book express a response to these changes in respect of the control of periodontal diseases. As caries has declined and dentate individuals have become more numerous, disorders of the periodontium have become of increasing concern to the general dental practitioner. These disorders require the practitioner to extend his traditional role as a skilled operator, so that he also becomes a counsellor, a motivator, a monitor and a team leader. For years dentists have been enjoined to adopt such roles but little or no guidance has been provided. At last here is a book which explains what needs to be done and how it should be done.

By building around the concept of using periodontal indices as tools of clinical measurement, the authors of this book provide a detailed blueprint describing the necessary attitudinal and management changes required to accomplish these new tasks. The approach adopted is entirely consistent with modern research findings and with the methods for the control of the periodontal diseases advocated most authoritatively by the World Health Organisation and the Federation Dentaire Internationale. If the text is carefully followed the dentist will discover simple systems for quantifying and recording the features of periodontal disease and will be able to make sensible interpretations of the data when taking clinical decisions. The importance of this unique book is that it offers to the dentist freedom from the uncertainty and frustration traditionally associated with the management of periodontal disease. Although Lewis Carroll, in his poem "Four Riddles", wrote:

> "Yet what are all such gaieties to me
> Whose thoughts are full of indices and
> surds?"

it does appear that exactly the opposite will be the case for the dentist who is prepared to develop new attitudes and to master the techniques described here.

R. Duckworth.

Introduction

It is currently believed that somewhere between 7 and 15% of the world population are highly susceptible to some form of destructive periodontal disease. Thus from a periodontal point of view every dental practitioner has a certain number of patients at risk, whatever his speciality and locality of practice. Perhaps of more significance, all other dental treatment, be it complex bridgework, prosthetics, orthodontics or day-to-day restorative work will be prone to failure in those patients if the periodontal problem is not managed effectively.

The importance of the problem to all dentists is clear. The solution however is not so easy. At the present time there are no satisfactory techniques to predict in advance of signs of the disease which patients belong to the high risk group. Furthermore, future diagnostic tests will probably be more concerned with systemic and microbiological factors: patients who develop the disease because of gross neglect of plaque control procedures or because of the development of localised plaque retentive factors will not be detected by such tests.

It seems therefore that present and future techniques of periodontal care will have to rely upon careful and quantitative assessment of disease features, particularly in the early stages. Based upon this premise we have endeavoured for some years to develop a flexible system of periodontal care which would be suitable for application in general dental practice and which would conform with current academic opinion.

This has not been easy however because of changes in the understanding of the disease process itself, and in the reactions of patients to various forms of therapy. It is now believed that periodontal diseases are site specific within the mouth, that individuals vary widely in response to aetiological factors and that the progression of the disease is episodic and may even be cyclical. All of these effects have to be taken into account when designing a system of periodontal care.

On the credit side we have been encouraged to pursue our goal by two recent developments. The first of these has been the sponsorship by the World Health Organisation and the International Dental Federation of one means of measuring periodontal disease, the Community Periodontal Index of Treatment Needs (CPITN). Whatever the future value of the CPITN as an epidemiological and manpower planning tool proves to be, the diagnostic aspects

9

of the system seem to be embraced easily by dentists for use as a periodontal screening system in individual patients.

The second development of interest is the publication by the British Society of Periodontology of a policy statement entitled "Periodontology in General Dental Practice in the United Kingdom". The document concerns itself with the problems outlined above and makes initial proposals which have the support of a wide cross-section of members of that Society.

We have encapsulated these developments into a Periodontal Control System which we consider to be easy for the general practitioner to apply to large numbers of patients despite the magnitude and complexity of the periodontal problem. However, as is the case with some things which are simple to carry out, the Periodontal Control System requires much explanation and justification before its full value is understood. This book, which is in no way intended to replace the several excellent texts on the general subject of periodontology, will show the value of the System and explain how to implement it in practice.

A.M. Grace, F.C. Smales.
October 1988

Tooth Numbering Systems

In the forms illustrated in this book, tooth number is indicated using the Palmer/Zsigmondy System commonly employed in the United Kingdom.

The advent of the International Tooth Numbering System (International Standards Organisation ISO 3950 (1984)) means that earlier numbering systems are superseded.

Consequently, the ISO tooth numbers have been added to the forms as appropriate and should be the only tooth numbers used in future.

PART I

THE CHANGING VIEW OF PERIODONTAL DISEASE

Our main aim in writing this book is to suggest a method of providing periodontal care which is appropriate for the general dental practitioner. We have found that the most satisfactory approach to this involves the understanding and use of a system of monitoring the patient's periodontal condition using indices. Because this procedure is unfamiliar to many practitioners we feel it is important to explain why we are giving indices such prominence.

Periodontology is one of the most rapidly-changing disciplines in dentistry and consequently great care is needed when proposing techniques of diagnosis, methods of assessing prognosis and therapy. Before looking in more detail at the use of indices in what we have called the Periodontal Control System we need to see how they relate to the way in which concepts central to periodontology have changed over the last two decades.

Chapter 1

The Nature of Periodontal Disease

The Traditional Approach

For many years the main attitude towards the nature of periodontal disease was based upon the following beliefs:

1. Periodontal disease was widespread throughout the world and affected 98% of the population (1).
2. Periodontal disease was a slow, steady process that gradually led to the inevitable loss of teeth in all patients (1, 2) unless halted in a single course of treatment.

Coupled with these attitudes was a further belief that treatment involved preparation of the mouth for periodontal surgery by scaling and plaque control techniques. The surgery would then remove the compromised tissues and enable the patient to clean more effectively. It was assumed that, following this surgery, the improved oral environment would favour plaque control procedures which would in turn prevent recurrence of the disease. This therapeutic concept is summarised in Fig. 1.1.

The Importance of Plaque

With the realisation of the importance of the role of plaque in the aetiology of the disease process (3) came a new approach to treatment which tended to result in a longer pre-operative phase during which an attempt was made to create the ideal, a plaque-free mouth. This approach improved the prognosis following periodontal surgery, but also resulted in the unexpected finding that some patients responded so well to

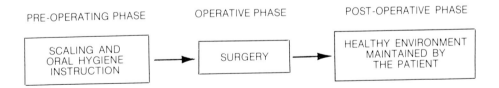

Fig. 1.1   The traditional concept of therapy.

plaque control alone that surgery was no longer needed. This model for periodontal care is displayed in Fig. 1.2.

This model of disease control is worthy of further consideration because it forms the key to much of the present thinking about periodontal care.

STEP 1: The patient is found to require periodontal treatment.

STEP 2: Plaque control instruction is provided.

STEP 3: If the patient's plaque control is inadequate, instruction is repeated until either the periodontal condition improves or the patient becomes disillusioned and seeks treatment elsewhere.

STEP 4: If the patient's plaque control is adequate the disease either resolves (in which case the patient is maintained and observed) or remains (in which case surgery is carried out).

Some Drawbacks

Although this approach was a great improvement on what had gone before, eventually drawbacks became apparent. The emphasis on the patient's ability to practise good plaque control as the deciding factor in therapy tended to create frustration for patients unable to cooperate fully.

When faced with a patient who appears unable to clean adequately the usual reaction of the dentist is to believe that the patient has failed to understand how to clean. More careful and detailed instruction is then given, as if the *provision* of the information alone is enough to cause behavioural change. If the patient does not then comply the dentist or hygienist does not know what to do next, except to repeat the information.

The patient's failure to comply with the new instructions however are often due not to lack of knowledge, but more to lack of motivation. They may know *how* to clean, but do not have good enough reasons *why* they should clean. This will be discussed more fully in Chapter 12. Another drawback in the plaque control model is the use of undefined terms such as "adequate control" and "inadequate control". This results in a situation where neither the general practitioner nor the patient know what is really required. A patient, working hard at cleaning and flossing, could still present with some plaque and be told that the level of plaque control was "inadequate" or "not good enough". It is hardly surprising that this rebuff could itself lead to a loss of motivation.

Attitudes to Treatment

In our opinion the most important (and least understood and recognised) factor contributing to the failure of periodontal therapy has been the attitude of the dentist or hygienist towards the way in which periodontal therapy is delivered.

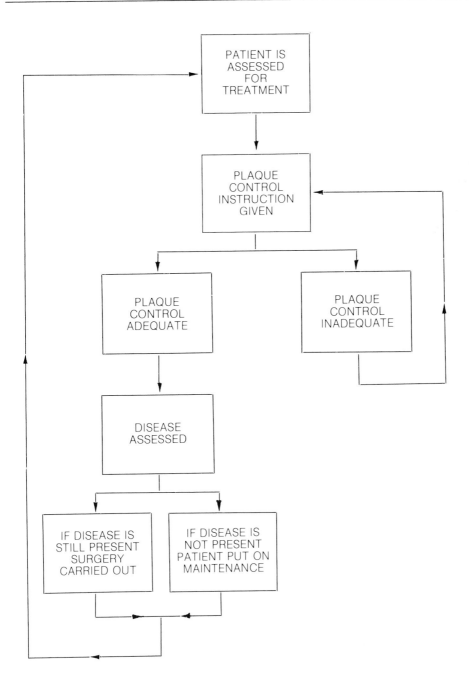

Fig. 1.2   The Plaque Control Model of Therapy.

Most dental treatment is provided as a "package", a closed unit of defined procedures that has a beginning (the examination), a middle (providing the filling, doing the crown preparation, taking impressions for the denture, etc.) and a definite end (fitting the denture, extracting the tooth). Then, as far as the patient (and dentist) is concerned, that treatment is complete. On a further visit it is unlikely that the denture or crown will need replacing but a new "package" of treatment may be started.

In the past a course of periodontal treatment has been considered to be a similar "package"; a closed unit of treatment (Fig. 1.3) which followed the same philosophy of thinking inherent in the provision of a filling or denture. First came the beginning (the examination), then the middle (the plaque control instruction and scaling) and finally the end (the surgical procedure), and upon removal of the pack and sutures treatment was complete. It is important to realise that it is the perception by the patient of the *fundamental attitude of the practitioner* that is being described here, not the reality.

The most striking feature of this perceived attitude towards periodontal treatment was the lack of emphasis on the importance of aftercare. Studies have shown this to be the main factor in determining long-term success or failure, particularly after periodontal surgery (4, 5). Even though the dentist or hygienist may talk about the importance of aftercare, should the fundamental approach to periodontal therapy be that of the "closed box", the patient's attitude

will be influenced so that treatment will tend to fail in the long-term.

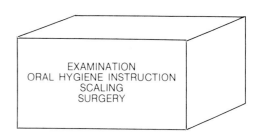

EXAMINATION
ORAL HYGIENE INSTRUCTION
SCALING
SURGERY

Fig. 1.3   The Closed Box Concept.

The Importance of Regular Visits

In the late 1970s there emerged a new concept of periodontal care (based on studies carried out in Scandinavia and the United States (6, 7, 8). These studies showed that patients making regular frequent visits at about 3-monthly intervals to dental centres, usually to be seen by a hygienist, showed a remarkable improvement in their periodontal condition compared with patients not undergoing the same programme.

The essence of these studies was that fairly large groups of people (often 200 – 500 patients) were split into equally divided groups; one group receiving "regular" dental care (they attended the dentist when they felt the need or were on a recall system) whilst the other group returned to see the hygienist on average every 3 months.

After a period of time (usually several years) the groups were reassessed to compare the difference in periodontal deterioration. The group being seen by the hygienist at 3-monthly intervals showed much improvement over the control group.

These results led to the realisation that in the longterm repeated visits for periodontal care had the following advantages:

1. The patients were more easily motivated because they developed a relationship with the dentist or hygienist.
2. The disease had less time to cause further and less easily reversed deterioration before the patient was seen again.
3. After surgery a system of aftercare was automatically initiated which tended to reduce failure of the surgery (4, 5).
4. Many problem areas which would previously have required surgery resolved with scaling and oral hygiene alone (9).

The most important change in attitude following these studies was the realisation that periodontal disease appears to need more frequent monitoring than is usually provided, especially within the framework of general practice.

The "Continuing Care" Concept

If we consider the "closed box" approach to treatment described earlier (Fig. 1.3) it can be seen that with the recognition of the importance of regular visits it becomes necessary to consider routine periodontal care as a large number of "boxes" (or units of treatment) given in frequent succession (Fig. 1.4). The last conceptual step required to arrive at the continuing care concept is to convert Fig. 1.4.a to Fig. 1.4.b where the succession of units is transformed into one continuous unit that has no end. Thus following the initial examination, consultations continue, albeit intermittently, as a series of visits of varying frequency for monitoring the situation and providing advice in plaque control and scaling where appropriate.

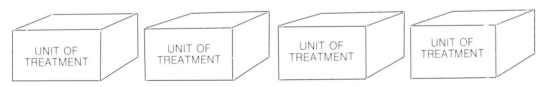

Fig. 1.4.a   A succession of units of treatment.

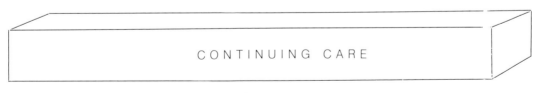

Fig. 1.4.b   The continuous care concept.

Although the jump from Fig. 1.4.a to Fig. 1.4.b may itself appear a small one if we are considering the content of the visits only, the shift in thinking required by both the dentist, hygienist and patient is much greater. The "closed unit" of treatment is so ingrained into all dental thinking (including the contractual single and complete course of treatment) that both patient and dentist find this change in attitude extremely difficult.

This problem was commented on by Kerr (4) when he attributed the failure of the periodontal surgery seen in patients referred back to their regular dentist to the lack of an adequate recall system within the practice. This important and often overlooked aspect will be covered in more detail in Chapter 10.

In order to provide a "continuing care" style of treatment it becomes necessary to find a structure which is easy to use and acceptable to all parties. Monitoring of patients by using indices, which can be recorded at every visit and explained to the patient when necessary, provides just such a structure.

The Dynamic Nature of the Disease

Coupled with this change in attitude towards periodontal therapy came the revelation that the progression and distribution of periodontal disease was not a slow, steady state of continuing deterioration throughout the mouth, but more a dynamic and cyclic disease affecting isolated areas at specific times to differing degrees.

Although this pattern had often been observed in individual patients it began to be considered seriously to represent the more generalised situation following papers in 1982 and 1983 (10, 11). In these studies patients had certain pocket depths measured on a monthly basis. No treatment was given, and the results showed that most pockets appeared to remain static and only a few (3-5%) changed depth significantly (2-5mm). Whilst some pockets deepened others improved, reinforcing the concept of a cyclic disease which, without therapy, could lead either to loss of attachment or to healing.

The Relevance of the "Burst" Theory of Disease Activity

If this model of disease activity is accepted then it should be apparent that regular treatment for a disease that is inactive is rather like treating a patient for influenza using the information that he has had an episode in the past and may suffer one again in the future.

The major difference in periodontal disease as opposed to influenza is that in the case of the latter the patient is well aware of his condition. Periodontal disease is so painless and insidious that the patient is unlikely to be aware of anything amiss until the damage is extensive.

Thus it becomes necessary for the dentist to keep a regular check (by using a system of indices) on the condition of the periodontal tissues to ensure that should a burst of activity affect any particular site the appropriate treatment can be initiated without delay.

Regular Monitoring

If the continuing care concept of periodontal therapy is combined with the dynamic and cyclic nature of disease activity then a definite pattern of periodontal care emerges which is of great significance to the practitioner.

Patients will require monitoring on a regular basis to ensure that the activity of the disease is static. Should an area of the mouth exhibit signs of disease activity then appropriate treatment procedures should be initiated until the disease activity slows down again, when routine monitoring should be restored.

At times of susceptibility to the disease process the patient will require more frequent care, whilst during periods of inactivity the intervals between monitoring visits can be lengthened. Should any surgical procedure be required, that procedure should be considered purely as an adjunct to the continuing care concept rather than an end in itself.

Summary

Past concepts of periodontal disease and its treatment have been discussed at some length. The old ideas of therapy have tended to revolve around several erroneous concepts, especially the fact that the disease is both widespread and inevitable. This has resulted in courses of treatment that concentrated on the idea of creating health by removal of the cause (plaque control) followed by removal of the diseased tissue (surgery). We have also described the change in awareness about the activity and progression of periodontal disease coupled with the evidence for the importance of regular visits. Combining these two ideas introduces a system of periodontal monitoring to the practitioner which has the following advantages:

1: It provides a quantitative view of the disease for a patient over a period of time.
2: It will indicate that a burst of activity of disease has taken place.
3: It provides information regarding the distribution of disease within the mouth.
4: It provides the patient with a worthwhile and personally relevant reason for attending regularly.
5: It gives a reliable method of assessing the success of therapy.

The other aspect of periodontal care which contributes to success is an understanding of the factors involved in motivating appropriate patient behaviour. These are particularly relevant in periodontal therapy as they control the wish of the patient to continue to seek care, and more importantly, to continue with an effective method of homecare. Monitoring plays an important role in motivation as well as in the measurement and control of therapy, as we shall show in Chapter 12.

References

1. W.H.O. (1978): Epidemiology, aetiology and prevention of periodontal diseases report of a W.H.O. Scientific Group. Technical report series no. 621. Geneva, World Health Organisation.
2. Loe H., Anerud A., Boysen H. & Smith M. (1978): The natural history of periodontal disease in man. The rate of periodontal destruction before 40 years of age. Journal of Periodontology 49 607-620.
3. Loe H., Theilade E., & Jensen S. B., (1965): Experimental gingivitis in man. Journal of Periodontoloy 36 177-187.
4. Kerr N.W. (1981): Treatment of chronic periodontitis. British Dental Journal 150 222-224.
5. Axelsson P. & Lindhe J., (1981): The significance of maintenance care in the treatment of periodontal disease. Journal of Clinical Periodontology 8 281-294.
6. Lovdal A., Arno A., Schei O. & Waerhaug J. (1961): Combined effect of subgingival scaling and controlled oral hygiene on the incidence of gingivitis. Acta Odont. Scand. 19 537-555.
7. Suomi J.D., Greene J.C., Vermillion J.R., et al (1971): The effect of controlled oral hygiene procedures on the progression of periodontal disease in adults. Journal of Periodontology 42 152-160.
8. Axelsson P. & Lindhe J. (1981): Effect of controlled hygiene procedures on caries and periodontal disease in adults – Results after 6 years. Journal of Clinical Periodontology 8 239-248.
9. Badersten A., Nilveus R. & Egelberg J. (1981): Effect of non-surgical periodontal therapy: 1. Moderately advanced periodontitis. Journal of Clinical Periodontology 8 57-72.
10. Goodson J.M., Tanner A.C.R., Haffajee A.D., Sornberger G.C. & Socransky S.S. (1982): Patterns of progression and regression of advanced destructive periodontal disease. Journal of Clinical Periodontology 9 472-481.
11. Socransky S.S., Haffajee A.D., Goodson J.M. & Lindhe J. (1984): New concepts of destructive periodontal disease. Journal of Clinical Periodontology 11 21-32.

PART 2

PERIODONTAL INDICES

In this section of the book we will concentrate on the skills required to enable the practitioner to provide a comprehensive periodontal control programme. These skills centre around the ability to record the diagnostic signs and symptoms of the disease using periodontal indices which have been adapted to facilitate their use in general practice.

It is not implied that these indices are suitable for use in research projects or epidemiological surveys, nor are we justifying their use on the basis of formal scientific evidence. We are simply proposing an alternative use of periodontal indices to suit the needs of general practice in much the same way that systematic examination and coding of the state of the teeth is used at present to help the practitioner plan restorative treatment for the patient.

The indices which we will consider record the basic signs of the disease, bleeding and loss of attachment as well as the level of plaque and we will concentrate upon the technique of determining individual indices. Periodontal treatment however involves much more than just monitoring and motivation. Complicated topics such as the complete diagnosis of disease, root planing, scaling, oral hygiene instruction, the pathology and immunology of the disease process and techniques of surgical procedures are involved. These are well covered in many textbooks but what is often omitted from other books is the practical reality of *planning the delivery of these items of care to provide a comprehensive periodontal control programme*. In the United Kingdom for example these considerations have to be related to the structure and financial constraints of the National Health Service. Elsewhere similar constraints of time and expense apply.

The Periodontal Control System is one approach to the delivery of care. In Part 3 the way in which indices are combined with one another and with additional clinical data to give a complete control system is described.

Chapter 2

Using the Community Periodontal Index of Treatment Needs in Practice

Until recently the general practitioner had no definite tool to aid in the assessment of the periodontal status of a patient other than clinical judgement. In the environment of general practice this made it much harder to diagnose the early signs of disease, and unless a rigorous and self-imposed discipline was carried out routinely on every patient it was possible to fail to identify many patients with the potential for periodontal destruction.

The situation has changed in the last few years with the development of an index which has been accepted internationally, the Community Periodontal Index of Treatment Needs (CPITN). We feel this index to be an extremely useful aid as a routine procedure for use with all patients which will enable the practitioner to identify those who require further investigation.

The Community Periodontal Index of Treatment Needs (CPITN)

One of the first decisions that the practitioner must make is whether the patient *needs* periodontal care, and if so how

much. Although it is possible to make an assessment using a combination of clinical experience and diagnosis, this approach suffers from subjective bias and also the very real possibility that isolated areas of periodontal destruction will have been overlooked. At the other extreme it is possible to use various indices to assess plaque levels, the presence or absence of bleeding and probing depths, but these steps are time-consuming and unnecessarily complex if at the end of assessment the patient's periodontal tissues are found to be healthy and not to require any further treatment.

The CPITN which has been sponsored by the World Health Organisation and the Federation Dentaire Internationale, is designed mainly as an indicator of treatment need (1). This index provides a rapid and reproducible method of assessing the periodontal condition of the patient *at the first visit*. The information acquired by using the CPITN can also be used to help the clinician decide which further indices are required as well as indicating probable treatment needs.

The WHO Probe

The CPITN relies entirely for its scoring on a special type of periodontal probe which was developed by the WHO solely for this index. The probe has 2 special characteristics which are mandatory for the collection of the CPITN, and which prevent it from being used for generalised probing depth measurements.

Firstly, it has a ball-ended tip of 0.5 mm diameter. Secondly, instead of the usual 1 or 2 mm graduations, there is a colour-coded band of 2 mm on the shaft beginning 3.5 mm from the tip (see Fig. 2.1).

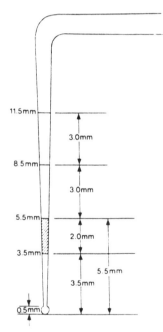

Fig. 2.1 The WHO Probe.

A further development of the probe incorporates two further gradations at 8.5 mm and 11.5 mm. We have not found this modification to be useful in our system.

The rationale for the ball-ended tip is two-fold. Firstly, detection of subgingival calculus is made easier. Secondly, excessive pressure by an inexperienced operator when using the probe is less likely to cause penetration of the tissues. The recommended probing force is between 15-25 grams, a surprisingly light force when contrasted with the more robust actions used with sharp diagnostic probes and other dental instruments. This important point will be discussed more fully in Chapter 5.

The first colour-coded band allows the operator to assess instantly whether the probing depth is less than 3.5 mm, between 3.5 and 5.5 mm, or in excess of 5.5 mm. These divisions are significant because they divide periodontal pockets into 3 classifications by depth which most periodontologists believe would respond best to different types of treatment.

Assessing the Index

The index is determined by using the probe to detect the presence or absence of:

1. Bleeding on probing.
2. Calculus or overhanging restorations.
3. Periodontal pockets.

In compiling this index the teeth and their associated periodontal units are divided into six groups or sextants. Although all surfaces of each standing tooth are examined only the worst periodontal unit in each sextant is recorded. Care is taken in young people to discount false pocketing on recently erupted teeth like the 3rd molars when assigning the sextant scores.

Four of the sextants are composed of the molars and premolars of each quadrant and two of the sextants contain the incisors and canines of the upper and lower jaws.

If only one tooth is present in a sextant its periodontal unit is included in the assessment of the adjacent sextant. For example if only 11 was present in the anterior sextant the score would be assessed with the remaining teeth in the upper right posterior sextant, whereas if 21 was the only anterior tooth present the score would be assessed with the upper left posterior sextant.

In children and adolescents (under 20 years) the official CPITN system recommends that the score is taken on 6 key teeth only as shown in Fig. 2.2 to avoid scoring false pockets which arise during the eruption of teeth. Experience from epidemiological studies also suggest that in such patients the presence of destructive disease around teeth other than the permanent molars and incisors is highly unlikely.

Examination of the patient is performed by passing the probe into the gingival sulcus of a tooth, ensuring that it is parallel with the long axis of that tooth. Care is taken to probe each interdental

16	11	26
46	31	36

Fig. 2.2 Key teeth recommended by CPITN System (patients under 20 years).

area and buccal and lingual surfaces. The operator should be alert for external signs of pocket formation, as trials show inexperienced operators commonly miss isolated deep pockets. Starting on one tooth the whole mouth is systematically examined. Scoring is performed as follows:

Code 4: The probe penetrates a pocket so that the whole of the coloured band disappears — indicating a pocket of 6mm or more.

Code 3: The probe penetrates a pocket so that only part of the coloured band is visible — indicating a pocket between 3.5mm and 5.5mm.

Code 2: The whole of the coloured band of the probe is visible but supra- or subgingival calculus or the defective margin of a filling or crown are detected — shallow pockets only.

Code 1: Bleeding elicited after gentle probing without calculus or pocketing being present.

Code 0: Healthy tissues.

In the BSP recommendations (3) note is taken during the screening procedure of furcations or excessive recession. An asterisk is suggested to replace the sextant score when a furcation can be probed, or when the total attachment loss at a site is 7mm or more.

Recording the Results

Once the worst score has been found in each sextant it is recorded on a grid similar to the one in Fig. 2.3.

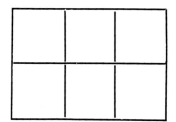

Fig. 2.3   The Grid used in the CPITN.

The main advantage of the CPITN is that it is a simple and rapid scoring system and can be added to a variety of charts with ease. The main disadvantage is that there is very little indication of the true severity of the problem for patients with scores of 3 or 4, as these could mean that only a single tooth in the sextant is involved or that every tooth has seriously damaged support. However, if use of the index is restricted to *identifying* patients requiring more extensive therapy who can then have more detailed and specific assessments it is a very useful aid. We regard it as extremely important to limit the use of the CPITN for individual patients to a preliminary assessment technique. In particular the 6 coded numbers must *never* be added or averaged in an attempt to provide a single figure to represent the periodontal condition of the whole mouth. This can be accomplished by using the Periodontal Index which is described in Chapter 6, although the resulting figure for an individual patient must be interpreted with great caution.

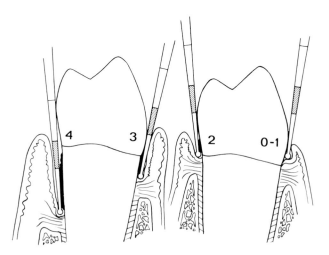

Fig. 2.4   Using the probe to determine the CPITN reading.

Summary

Patients who require more extensive periodontal investigation and care in general practice can be identified by using a simple, reproducible index that can be recorded routinely for every patient.

One such index, the CPITN, has been described. Although this index was primarily developed for epidemiological purposes it can readily be adapted for general practice use (2). There are advantages to having an index which can be recorded as a routine screening method on every patient and the results used to identify those patients requiring further periodontal investigation.

Our own interpretation of the scoring system will be presented fully in Chapter 7.

References

1. Ainamo J., Barmes D., Beagrie G., Cutress, T., Martin J., & Sardo-Infirri, J. (1982): Development of the World Health Organisation Community Periodontal Index of Treatment Needs. International Dental Journal 32, 281-291.
2. Croxson L.J. (1984): A simplified periodontal screening examination: the Community Perio-dontal Index of Treatment Needs (WHO) in general practice. International Dental Journal 34 28-34.
3. Periodontology in General Practice in the United Kingdom: A First Policy Statement. The British Society of Periodontology May 1986.

Chapter 3

The Relevance of Plaque

Having selected those patients who require some periodontal treatment by use of the CPITN (see Chapter 2) together with clinical judgement, it is necessary to categorise patients into:

* those who require complex treatment.
* those who require simple treatment.
* those who fall somewhere between.

One advantage of the CPITN is that when used to detect disease and its associated features the scoring system provides a ready-made classification which can be used in treatment planning. In brief, any patient with codes 3, 4 or * in one or more sextants can be considered as probably requiring complex treatment, subject to further investigation. Patients with no Codes 3, 4 or * but with Code 2 in 2 or more sextants would be borderline, whilst patients with Code 1 only or Code 2 in a single sextant could be considered as requiring simple treatment only. Those patients with scores of 0 in all sextants will require no treatment, but will need to be recalled for a CPITN screening examination in one year's time. This will be expanded in Part 3 of the book.

After mutual decisions are made by patient and practitioner regarding whether and how to proceed with further diagnosis and treatment, the CPITN has to be supplemented with additional indices. This is because using the CPITN after initial screening to provide the sole baseline and monitoring data has disadvantages, the most significant of these being the lack of response by the index to the effects of early therapy. In other words although the patient may make substantial improvements in plaque control causing the inflammatory reaction in many periodontal units to show a corresponding reduction, the CPITN could show exactly the same scores as those seen initially because one or two periodontal units in each sextant had failed to respond.

The patient is best served then if we use an index that will respond with a reduction as soon as the patient improves cleaning, so we can detect the change and reinforce it by encouragement. Because the CPITN is linked to probing depths, bleeding and calculus instead of plaque it may take several weeks before any dramatic change is likely to be measurable, and it is entirely possible that the patient will have lost interest by then.

To advance the treatment planning process further and in particular to enable us to measure any improvement in plaque control we need an index that measures plaque, and in particular that plaque which is susceptible to the removal techniques used by the patient.

The Role of Plaque

There is now such overwhelming evidence for the implication of dental plaque in the initiation and progression of periodontal disease, albeit sometimes in a more complicated form than previously believed, that we do not need to make further comment here. Although the exact mechanisms involved often remain obscure it is generally accepted that plaque initiates an inflammatory reaction within the tissues of the gingivae resulting in a gingivitis, which in some cases may progress to a periodontitis. Whether this is due to a change in the bacterial flora, a weakening in the immune response, or direct bacterial invasion of the tissues is still not clear. At the clinical level most patients suffer from a gingival reaction to plaque, usually in the form of inflammation. If the plaque is removed regularly the tissues heal and the periodontium is restored to health. Yet in some patients continuous exposure to high plaque levels appears to cause very little reaction so the signs of disease are extremely few or even absent altogether. Conversely in other patients minimal amounts of plaque are responsible for extensive gingival and periodontal damage.

These last two extremely different reactions to plaque are however the opposing ends of a continuous scale of varying response. Most patients fall somewhere at or near the midway point, experiencing some periodontal damage in response to plaque. For these patients plaque control practised on a regular basis is often sufficient to keep the disease from progressing.

Methods of Plaque Measurement

There are four basic approaches to the measurement of plaque:-

1. Collection of the plaque (using instruments such as scalers) which is then weighed or estimated chemically to calculate the amount. This is obviously impractical in practice.

2. Methods which estimate the *thickness* of plaque, usually on the crown of the tooth near the gingival margin. These methods can give rise to difficulty because of lack of agreement over the degree of thickness between individual operators. Such difficulties would suggest that an index based on plaque thickness is unsuitable for use in general practice alalthough it remains the method of choice in clinical trials where ideally a single individual takes the score.

3. Methods which estimate the *area* of plaque covering the crown of the tooth (see Fig. 3.1). These indices are easier for dentist and hygienist to estimate and in our hands have shown an acceptable consistency between dentists and hygienists after minimal training, thus making them acceptable for general practice.

4. Methods which measure the presence or absence of plaque on teeth.

Although simple to perform these indices tend to be fairly time-consuming, and may fail to change in response to early improvements in plaque control. They do, however, have value in the motivation of certain patients, so compensating in those cases for the extra effort of dentist or hygienist.

Choice of Plaque Index

The choice of plaque index depends upon the *reason* for taking the index. As we have already mentioned any form of index for use in general practice needs to be:

    simple to perform
    quick to do
    easy to record
    comprehended by the patient
    reproducible by different dentists and
        hygienists

The other important feature is that the index needs to detect an improvement in plaque levels even if the patient has only improved their oral hygiene marginally. The detection of such improvement is very relevant in the process of behaviour change discussed in Chapter 1 and expanded in Part 4.

Of the 4 methods mentioned above only the last 2 can be considered as suitable for general practice, and both will be discussed.

The Debris Index

The Debris Index (D.I.) is based on the debris index (simplified) of Greene and Vermillion (1) and measures the *area* of the tooth covered by plaque (Fig. 3.1). The D.I. is taken by measuring the amount of plaque covering the surfaces of 6 selected teeth, usually after disclosing. The amount of plaque is scored as below:

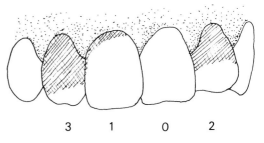

Fig. 3.1   Scoring for the Debris Index.

Grade 0: No plaque on the tooth.

Grade 1: Plaque covering up to one third of the surface.

Grade 2: Plaque covering more than one third but less than two thirds of the tooth surface.

Grade 3: Plaque covering more than two thirds of the tooth surface.

The clinical technique involves disclosing all the teeth in as uniform a fashion as possible. We usually recommend the patient chews a disclosing tablet, circulates the resulting coloured saliva around the mouth and rinses out. The buccal and palatal surfaces (including the visible mesial and distal portions on each side of the tooth) are then examined for stained plaque.

This disclosing is for the purposes of scoring the index only and not for demonstrating the plaque to the patient. As it is done frequently for some patients it must be socially acceptable. This means that blue-staining tablets should be avoided and that red stains should be rinsed away as much as possible before the end of the appointment.

The index has the advantage of requiring only a few representative teeth to be scored, (known as partial scoring) and gives values closely related to those obtained by looking at the whole mouth. The teeth most suitable for this purpose are often referred to as Ramfjord's teeth (2) and are as follows:

16	21	24
44	41	36

A refinement of the index includes running a blunt periodontal probe *just* within the gingival sulcus of both buccal and palatal sides of each representative tooth. If the tip of the probe collects some sulcular plaque (even though the tooth is otherwise plaque-free) a score of 1 is still recorded. Although this may seem harsh, plaque within the sulcus is potentially very damaging, and when present has to be detected by the scoring system.

As will be seen in Chapter 4 this procedure of running the probe in the sulcus also allows the operator to record the Bleeding Index at the same time, which is of great practical value with regard to saving time.

If each tooth has 2 scores (1 for the buccal and 1 for the palatal) then a total of 12 scores will be recorded (as in Fig. 3.2). An average is then obtained which becomes the D.I. for that visit.

One point to note is that the term "debris" is used because any form of "plaque" index tends to refer to the method of Silness and Loe (3) based on the *thickness* concept of measurement.

DI & BI SCORES

TOOTH	SURFACE	DI	BI
6⌋ (16)	buccal	2	
	lingual	2	
L⌊ (21)	buccal	1	
	lingual	1	
L4 (24)	buccal	0	
	lingual	1	
⌈6 (36)	buccal	2	
	lingual	3	
⌉7 (41)	buccal	1	
	lingual	1	
4⌉ (44)	buccal	1	
	lingual	2	
TOTAL SCORE		17	
INDEX		1.4	

Fig. 3.2 *This chart is used to calculate the Debris Index. The teeth to be scored are noted in the lefthand column and then the scores for the buccal and lingual of each tooth are recorded. These are then added together to give a total score which when divided by 12 gives the average. This figure (1.4) is the index.*

The Plaque Distribution Chart

The other method of recording plaque that is suitable for general practice involves scoring the *presence* or *absence* of plaque throughout the mouth (4). Once again the teeth are disclosed, and then if any plaque is present on the buccal, mesial, distal or palatal surface of each tooth a cross (or similar mark) is placed on a grid (see Fig. 3.3).

The main disadvantage of this type of score is the time required. One other important difference is the lack of immediate response to oral hygiene. Imagine the situation if the patient presents with several areas where more than one third of the tooth surface has plaque (Fig. 3.4). If plaque control is improved so that most of these areas become less than one third, then the D.I. score would reduce (see Fig. 3.4). Obviously in these circumstances the dentist or hygienist would compliment the patient on their success and thereby reinforce their behaviour. Under the same conditions the distribution chart will show little or no difference in score, as the distribution chart only records presence or absence of plaque and takes no account of amount.

The plaque distribution chart can play an important role in the patient with advanced rapid periodontal deterioration where knowledge of the distribution of plaque is more helpful.

Limitations of the Debris Index

Although the D.I. provides a quick, easy method of assessing the amount of plaque on the teeth (and hence the patient's ability to remove it) in certain situations the partial scoring system may mask areas of the mouth which give

PLAQUE DISTRIBUTION

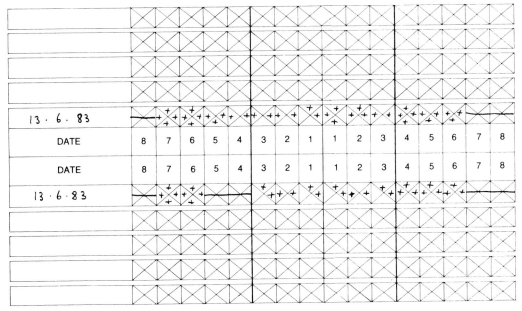

Fig. 3.3 On this chart each square represents a tooth divided into 4 sections, buccal, lingual, mesial and distal. A cross in the appropriate section signifies that plaque has been found in that section. This form of recording plaque does not distinguish between very small deposits and virtually total coverage.

an unrepresentative score. Thus a D.I. of 0.6 may represent significant achievement by the patient but hide the fact that for example the lower left molar region is particularly difficult for the patient and needs special attention.

This is an excellent example of the fact that indices only add to the traditional diagnostic skills of the dentist and do not

Summary

Plaque control has a central role in periodontal care, so a system of measuring plaque is required which gives an indication of the patient's individual reaction to plaque and the patient's response to plaque control instruction. Several different methods of measuring

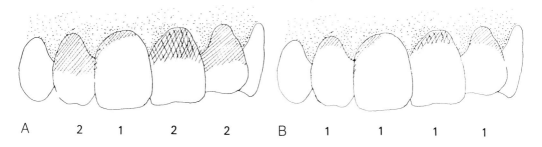

| A | 2 | 1 | 2 | 2 | B | 1 | 1 | 1 | 1 |

Fig. 3.4 On a plaque distribution chart the score would be the same for both (A) and (B) but on a D.I. score there would be an obvious reduction for (B).

supplant them. All the indices described in this book must be used intelligently as part of a diagnostic process.

In our experience of using the Debris Index the situation described above tends to be the exception however, and providing the operator is aware of possible limitations, the D.I. still remains one of the most effective methods of monitoring patient compliance with plaque control instructions over a period of time.

plaque have been discussed, and we are of the opinion that for general use in dental practice a simple method of measuring the area of plaque on 6 representative teeth is the best. The Debris Index provides just such an index, and is easy to learn, apply and record in practice.

We will be discussing the interpretation of the relationship of the D.I. to other indices in further chapters.

References

1. Greene J.C. & Vermillion J.R., (1964): The simplified oral hygiene index. Journal of the American Dental Association 68, 7-13.
2. Ramfjord S.P. (1959): Indices for prevalence and incidence of periodontal disease. Journal of Periodontology 30 51-59.
3. Silness J. & Loe H., (1963): Periodontal disease in pregnancy II: Correlation between oral hygiene and periodontal conditions. Acta Odontologica Scandinavica 22, 121-135.
4. O'Leary, T.J., Drake, R.B. & Naylor, J.E. (1972): The plaque control record. Journal of Periodontology 43 38.

Chapter 4

The Relevance of Bleeding

Gingival bleeding is often the only symptom of periodontal disease and bleeding on probing may well be the initial sign that alerts the clinician. It is also apparent that measurement of plaque alone is a poor basis for deciding the need for treatment, and an index such as the CPITN is preferable because it disregards the cause of the disease (plaque) and concentrates on the signs only (bleeding and pocket depths).

Another point to consider is that the Debris Index *by itself* will only provide information on the patient's ability to achieve and maintain good plaque control. To use this information effectively, particularly for those patients who have the initial stages of the disease, we need to make a comparison with an index of appropriate pathology, such as a bleeding index.

The Development of the Bleeding Index

There have been many indices used in the past to measure gingival inflammation, notably the PMA Index of Schour and Massler (1947) and the Gingival Index of Loe and Silness (1963)(1). One of the main difficulties of using these indices in practice has been the necessity to grade inflammation by using the colour and swelling characteristics of the marginal gingivae, a method open to different interpretation by different assessors. To one person red inflamed gingivae may appear healthy, to another diseased.

Originally the Gingival Index contained the rather vague term "bleeding on pressure" as part of the narrative, and although bleeding on pressure was later changed to bleeding on probing (2) there was still a necessity to estimate initial inflammation based on redness and swelling alone. In 1971 Muhlemann & Son overcame this by describing the Sulcus Bleeding Index (S.B.I.) which relied *entirely* on the presence of bleeding for an initial score and then incorporated colour and swelling into higher scores (3). This was later simplified by Cowell et al. in 1975 to a Bleeding Index which relies entirely on bleeding and ignores the other parameters of inflammation (4)

Grade 0   No bleeding on blunt probing
Grade 1   Bleeding on blunt probing up to 30 seconds later
Grade 2   Immediate bleeding on blunt probing
Grade 3   Spontaneous bleeding

In the general practice environment such an index has many advantages. It is quick to record, (using the teeth selected for the Debris Index), and easy to interpret as scoring relies solely on the presence or absence of bleeding. Furthermore, it is less likely to suffer from differences in scoring where a dentist and hygienist are working together than systems relying on colour and swelling.

Recording the Bleeding Index

The Bleeding Index uses partial-scoring as in the Debris Index, using the Ramfjord PDI teeth.

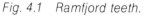

16		21	24
44	41		36

Fig. 4.1   Ramfjord teeth.

A blunt periodontal probe is used, and must be inserted just into the gingival sulcus first into the buccal then lingual side of each index tooth. The probe is then gently moved from mesial to distal within the sulcus without applying apical pressure. In other words the probe runs along the sulcus and not down into the depths of any pocket.

This is a variation on the recommendation of Cowell and his co-workers who specify probing to the base of any pocket (4). Bleeding from the depths of pockets in the Periodontal Control System is noted at the time of making probing depth measurement as described below. If there is any bleeding either immediately or up to 30 seconds later the appropriate score of 2 (for immediate bleeding) or 1 (for delayed bleeding) is recorded. If no bleeding occurs by 30 seconds a score of 0 is recorded.

When recording the Bleeding Index each of the index teeth is examined separately. The technique involves placing the tip of a blunt periodontal probe into the gingival sulcus mesially on the buccal surface of the tooth being examined and gently moving the probe to the distal of the tooth, keeping the tip just within the sulcus throughout the procedure. Immediate bleeding would be apparent. The probe can then be inserted into the palatal or lingual sulcus of the same tooth and the procedure repeated.

The operator can then return to examine the buccal surface visually to see if delayed bleeding has occurred before moving to the next index tooth. Similarly the palatal or lingual surface can be examined visually during the recording procedure on the next index tooth to check for delayed bleeding.

As mentioned in Chapter 3 one of the main advantages of using the Debris and Bleeding Indices together is that they can be recorded simultaneously. In order to check for sulcular plaque a periodontal probe needs to be inserted into the gingival sulcus and moved from mesial to distal. Exactly the same action is required to detect gingival bleeding. Thus the dentist or hygienist can assess both plaque and bleeding in the one movement.

The method of calculating the Bleeding Index is exactly the same as for the Debris Index. If each tooth has 2 scores (1 for the buccal and 1 for the palatal gingiva) then a total of 12 scores will be recorded (as in Fig. 4.2). An average is then obtained and this becomes the B.I. for the mouth at that visit.

DI & BI SCORES

TOOTH	SURFACE	DI	BI
6⌋ (16)	buccal		0
	lingual		1
l⌊ (21)	buccal		0
	lingual		0
l4 (24)	buccal		1
	lingual		2
⌈6 (36)	buccal		2
	lingual		2
7⌉ (41)	buccal		0
	lingual		1
4⌉ (44)	buccal		0
	lingual		2
TOTAL SCORE			11
INDEX			0·9

Fig. 4.2   This chart is used to calculate the Bleeding Index. The teeth to be scored are noted in the left-hand column and then the scores for the buccal and lingual of each tooth are recorded. These are then added together to give a total score – which when divided by 12 gives the average. This figure (0.9) is the index.

The Bleeding Points Chart

The Bleeding Points Chart records the distribution of bleeding around the mouth in the same way as the Plaque Distribution Chart. Although its compilation is time-consuming, this disadvantage can

BLEEDING POINTS DISTRIBUTION

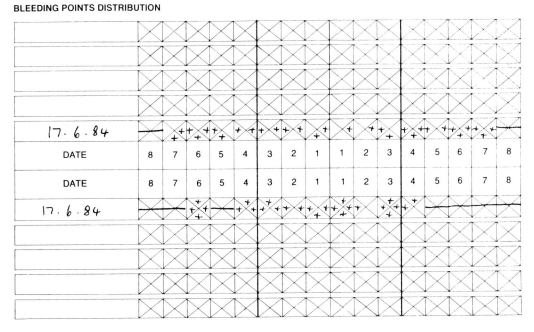

Fig. 4.3   On this chart each square represents a tooth divided into 4 sections, buccal, lingual, mesial and distal. A cross in the appropriate section signifies that blunt probing has elicited bleeding. This form of recording bleeding does not distinguish between bleeding at the depth of the pocket or gingival bleeding.

be minimised by measuring bleeding points at the same time as probing depths. Details of how much pressure to apply and the diameter of the probe used are covered in Chapter 5. Once the pockets have been probed a cross can be placed in the appropriate area on a distribution chart (as in Fig. 4.3) when bleeding occurs, whether it is delayed or immediate.

It is worth pointing out that in this example the Bleeding Point scores were collected as an extra procedure on the basis that the extra effort would be rewarded by the motivational effect it would achieve. Generally, this would not be performed for patients with superficial disease, and only occasionally for patients with more extensive disease.

BLEEDING POINTS DISTRIBUTION

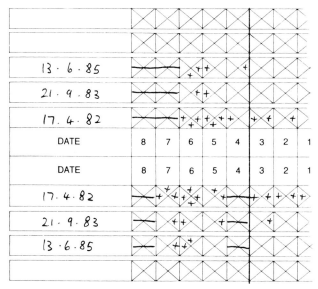

Fig. 4.4 On this chart the area between the upper right molars and the lower right molars is still bleeding on probing after three years, whereas most other areas appear to have resolved.

The advantages of such a chart are that:

1. It aids in the assessment of areas of particular concern identified by persistant bleeding over a period of time (Fig. 4.4).

2. It helps in patient motivation, especially if the patient can see a reduction in bleeding in one area of the mouth where particular emphasis has been placed on careful cleaning (as in Fig. 4.5).

This last point is of such practical value in aiding patients who have difficulty in flossing that we will discuss it in more detail. Fig. 4.5 shows a patient with generalised bleeding throughout the mouth on his first visit. He was encouraged to use dental floss interdentally between the lower incisors only until he had begun to form a habit. At the next visit approximately 2 weeks later he was shown the chart indicating a dramatic reduction in scoring (and hence

BLEEDING POINTS DISTRIBUTION

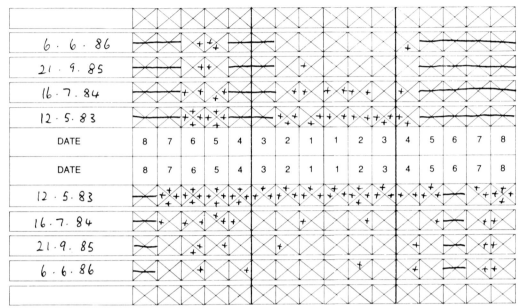

		8	7	6	5	4	3	2	1	1	2	3	4	5	6	7	8
6 · 6 · 86																	
21 · 9 · 85																	
16 · 7 · 84																	
12 · 5 · 83																	
DATE		8	7	6	5	4	3	2	1	1	2	3	4	5	6	7	8
DATE		8	7	6	5	4	3	2	1	1	2	3	4	5	6	7	8
12 · 5 · 83																	
16 · 7 · 84																	
21 · 9 · 85																	
6 · 6 · 86																	

Fig. 4.5 This chart indicates that, after twelve months, the lower anterior region has shown the most improvement to bleeding on probing. This is the area that the patient tends to floss regularly, and reinforces the link between using dental floss and prevention of disease.

bleeding) in the lower anterior region, where the floss had been used. This fact was shown to the patient and underlined the efficiency of floss, which in turn led to an enhanced desire on the part of the patient to start flossing elsewhere in an attempt to eliminate the remainder of the bleeding.

Difficulties in Interpretation

Bleeding is perhaps the most difficult sign to interpret for the inexperienced operator, and initial variations in scoring may lead to the belief that it is unreliable. It is important to remember that bleeding scores may lag behind plaque scores, so that an improvement in oral hygiene may not be reflected in a reduction in the Bleeding Index for several weeks or even longer. It is also possible that the dentist and hygienist may determine the Bleeding Index on the same day and record different values due to alterations in the gingival environment caused by the first probing.

Another point is that bleeding is an indicator of the phase of the disease at the time of measurement rather than representing the average state of the patient. Thus the trend of scores over a period of time is of more value than an isolated score.

Perhaps the most important guidance

provided by the Bleeding Index is when a patient with previously good plaque scores suddenly shows an increase in bleeding for no apparent reason (Fig. 4.6).

One interpretation of this finding is that a sudden burst of disease activity has occurred, or that susceptibility to the disease has increased. If the latter is true then a patient with existing good plaque control exhibiting such an increased susceptibility might benefit from extra help in the form of more frequent visits for professional plaque control procedures.

Summary

Bleeding is an early manifestation of periodontal disease for both patient and clinician. It is also a feature of gingival inflammation that is easy to record. As such it is an ideal indicator of the *reaction* of the patient to the aetiological factors present and subsequent therapy. The Bleeding Index is a simple, effective and relevant index for use in general practice and, fortunately can be recorded at the same time as the Debris Index. As such it is ideal as a complement to plaque scoring for routine use in general practice.

A Bleeding Points Chart is a valuable adjunct for the more susceptible patient. Because it involves little extra clinical time if probing depths are being recorded it is a valuable addition to the techniques of periodontal monitoring, both as an aid to motivation and as a record of the oral situation.

INITIAL TREATMENT

Date	DI	BI
16 · 1 · 92	0 · 9	0 · 3
23 · 3 · 82	0 · 6	0 · 2
17 · 8 · 82	0 · 4	0 · 1
2 · 3 · 83	0 · 3	0
11 · 11 · 83	0 · 4	0
6 · 7 · 84	0 · 4	0 · 7

Fig. 4.6 *This chart is a record of the debris index and bleeding index over a period of two and a half years. Whilst the D.I. has improved at the last visit the relatively high B.I. score suggests that this patient may require special attention as there appears to be an increase in disease susceptibility without a corresponding increase in plaque levels.*

References

1. Loe H. & Silness J. (1963): Periodontal disease in pregnancy I: Prevalence and severity. Acta Odontologica Scandinavica 21 533-551.
2. Loe H. (1967): The Gingival Index, the Plaque Index and the Retention Index systems. Journal of Periodontology 38 610-616.
3. Muhlemann H.R. & Son, S. (1971): Gingival sulcus bleeding – a leading symptom in initial gingivitis. Helvetia Odontologica Acta 15 107-113.
4. Cowell C.R., Saxton C.A., Sheiham A. and Wagg B.J. (1975): Testing therapeutic measures for controlling gingivitis procedures in man: a suggested protocol. Journal of Clinical Periodontology 2 231-240.

Chapter 5

Probing the Depths

Probably the most time-honoured measurement used in periodontology is the measurement of pocket depths, today called probing depths. In the past the *depth* of the pocket has been used to assess whether the disease is responding to therapy, and although there is evidence that pocket depth alone remains a poor indicator for treatment need, in the absence of a better alternative it still plays an important role in the overall assessment of periodontal disease progression.

Clinical Considerations

The main points to note about probing depth measurements can be summarised as:

1. The type of probe.
2. The force applied.
3. The angle of the probe.
4. The sites around the tooth.
5. The importance of recession.

Let us consider each of these in turn.

The Type of Probe

Because of the variety of probes available it is vital to select a single pattern that both the dentist and hygienist will use to ensure continuity in recording.

Recently various authorities have suggested that the best probe for general use is a Williams probe (Fig. 5.1) because the markings are irregularly spaced at 1, 2, 3, 5, 7, 8, 9 and 10mm intervals.

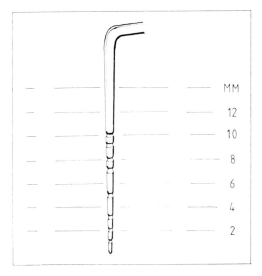

Fig. 5.1   A Williams Probe.

At first sight these variable intervals may appear confusing, but as the probe tip disappears into a deep pocket it is easier to establish the depth of penetration by observing the larger gap between 3-5mm or 5-7mm than to have to count the number of gradations as the probe is withdrawn. This is best understood by actually using the probe, but we will attempt an explanation as follows.

If one of the 2mm gaps is visible above the gingival margin then the probe has penetrated between 3 and 5mm, if both the 2mm gaps are visible the probe has penetrated 3mm or less, and if neither is visible the depth of the pocket is 7mm or over. In some ways this principle is similar to the coloured band on the CPITN probe discussed in Chapter 2.

The other important feature of the probe is the tip diameter. The World Health Organisation has recommended for the CPITN probe a tip of 0.5mm diameter and this is now becoming the accepted norm.

The Force Applied

The correct force to apply during probing depth measurements is obviously critical for correct diagnostic and follow-up recordings. With too much force the tip will penetrate the connective tissue (1). With too little the probing depth will be underestimated. The recommended force is 25 grams, and one way to calibrate oneself is to place the probe on a letter balance and press until the scales read 25 grams.

Recently a constant-force probe has been designed which will not allow a force in excess of a specified value to be applied (2). At present the probe is available giving 3 forces, 13 grams, 26 grams and 57 grams, and in our view use of this probe is an excellent way of ensuring accuracy as well as learning the correct pressure.

The Angle of the Probe

It is important to align the probe along the long axis of the tooth to ensure accurate and consistent results (Fig. 5.2).

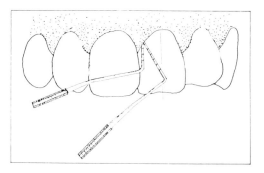

Fig. 5.2   The angle of the probe.

The Sites Around the Tooth

Measurement is usually taken at 6 different sites around each tooth (Fig. 5.3). This supplies data giving an overall picture of the periodontal situation throughout the mouth.

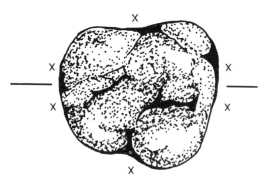

Fig. 5.3   Sites to take probing depths.

It is possible to restrict the recordings t 4 sites only around each tooth, taking the worst depth buccally or lingually at the mesial and distal parts of the tooth. However, as this still entails measuring mesially and distally it would seem better to record all 6 sites on the chart.

The Importance of Measuring Recession

The importance of measuring recession is often overlooked. Figure 5.4 shows a progressive loss of attachment *without any increase in pocket depth* which would lead to the assumption (based on probing depths alone) that no damage

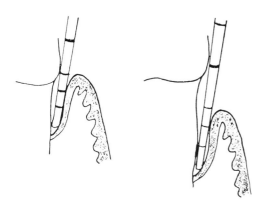

Fig. 5.4   The relevance of recession.

was occurring. Because the whole gingival unit is moving apically there is no deepening of the pocket and thus no obvious sign of progressing disease.

Recording the Information

Although measurement of probing depths is a reasonably standardised procedure there are many different styles of charting systems. Whichever system the practitioner chooses to adopt it should fulfil the following criteria:

1. The chart should be easy to read.
2. It should be simple to enter data.
3. Follow-up recordings should be entered on the same page.
4. There must be provision for recession recordings.
5. A pictorial representation is a valuable aid.

There are advantages to using a chart such as Fig. 5.5 which can be kept as a permanent record in the notes. This type of record sheet is extremely useful in motivating the patient, is useful for treatment planning, and can be a valuable record for medico-legal purposes.

Fig. 5.5 This probing depth chart has the following features:

1. *The mouth has been divided into sextants. Thus the only areas that need probing depths measured are those scoring 3 or 4 using the CPITN.*

2. *The measurements for recession have needed adjustment (following surgery in this case).*

3. *The pictorial representation is not intended to be accurate, but to allow the operator to see areas that require attention immediately without having to search through a mass of figures.*

Note that when the recession, probing depth or mobility is zero this is still scored to ensure that on future reference it is certain that the measurement was taken and recorded. An area measured zero but left blank could be interpreted as indicating that no measurement was recorded at all.

It is also important for the operator to check that sextants not measured at the commencement of treatment are still checked using the CPITN at a later date in case disease should start in that sextant.

Periodontal Control System

PROBING DEPTH CHART

NAME **MR J. JONES**   AGE **32 34 37**

BUCCAL (upper) — R ... L

2mm

	DATE															
RECESSION	23.7.82	—	13	14		2	10	11	01	10	3	—	2		0
POCKET DEPTH	23.7.82	—	246	832		235	722	426	523	444	668	—			
	23.1.84	—	227	722		224	623	335	632	222	458	—			
	1.10.84	—	228	822		222	422	225	622	222	348	—			
	3.12.85	—	223	323		222	122	211	212	122	213	—			
	23.4.86	—	222	212		212	222	223	422	122	214	—			
MOBILITY	23.7.82	—	1	2		0	0	0	0	0	1				
	1.10.84	—	0	0		0	0	0	0	0	0	—			
	23.4.86	—	0	0		0	0	0	0	0	0	—			

PALATAL — R ... L

2mm

	DATE														
RECESSION	23.7.82	—	02	02		0	0	0	0	0	0		0		0
POCKET DEPTH	23.7.82	—	447	964		444	643	326	544	444	510	—			
	23.1.84	—	237	1054		222	423	225	522	322	2310	—			
	1.10.84	—	227	1042		222	222	226	722	222	229	—			
	3.12.85	—	223	422		212	212	212	322	232	222	—			
	23.4.86	—	222	222		212	212	224	422	232	222	—			

LINGUAL — R ... L

2mm

	DATE												
RECESSION	23.7.82	0	0	0	—	0			0	0	0		
POCKET DEPTH	23.7.82	222	342	344	—	122			232	232	454		
	23.1.84	223	332	223	—	121			212	212	444		
	1.10.84	222	221	223	—	111			121	212	222		
	3.12.85	212	212	213	—	111			111	121	122		
	23.4.86	111	111	211	—	101			111	111	112		

BUCCAL (lower) — R ... L

2mm

	DATE															
RECESSION	23.7.82	2	2	2	—	3	2	0	0	0	0	2	0	0	2
POCKET DEPTH	23.7.82	223	222	223	—	212						222	232	425	
	23.1.84	222	232	223	—	212						122	222	444	
	1.10.84	222	222	222	—	212						212	222	223	
	3.12.85	222	212	112	—	111						111	212	112	
	23.4.86	212	212	111	—	111						111	212	112	
MOBILITY	23.7.82	0	0	0	—	0						0	0	0	
	1.10.84	0	0	0	—	0						0	0	0	
	23.4.86	0	0	0	—	0						0	0	0	

A Suggested Procedure

The actual method of recording information depends on the chart used, but the following steps improve efficiency and aid the D.S.A. in her recording.

1. First any missing teeth in the mouth should be marked on the

dontal probe midline buccally or lingually and measuring the distance (if any) between the cemento-enamel junction and the gingival margin (Fig. 5.7).

Gingival hyperplasia can be recorded by using a plus before the figure thus indicating "reverse recession" (or swelling).

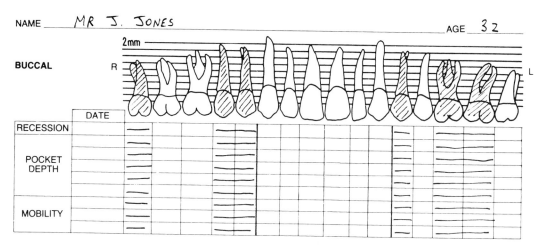

PROBING DEPTH CHART

Periodontal Control System

NAME _MR J. JONES_   AGE _32_

Fig. 5.6 The first stage in recording probing depths is to identify and mark out the missing teeth and the corresponding columns.

chart (Fig. 5.6). This is an essential step as the speed of the recording process relies in part on the dentist calling out figures rapidly and the D.S.A. being able to record them accurately and quickly in the correct place.

2. The next step is to record the recession around each tooth. This can be measured by placing the perio-

3. It is often best for the dentist to pause either at the midline or at the junction of each sextant to ensure that the D.S.A. is recording the correct information in the correct box on the chart. If a mistake has occurred then it is easier to correct it at this stage rather than discover it after all the probing depths have been identified.

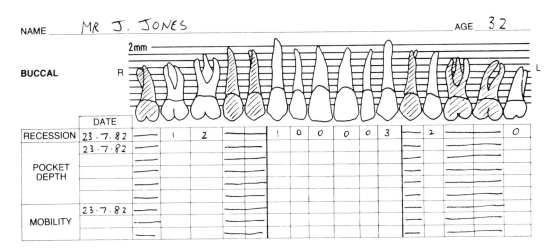

Fig. 5.7   *The next stage in recording probing depths is to write the date in the recession, pocket depth and mobility rows. The recession data is placed for all teeth regardless of the CPITN score.*

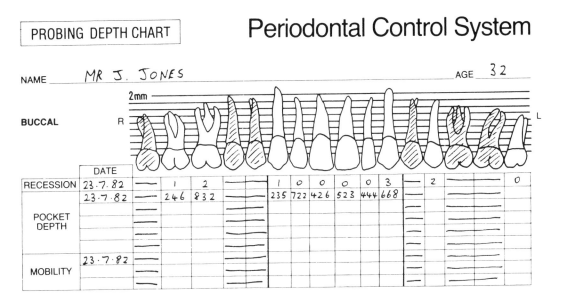

Fig. 5.8   *The next stage in recording probing depths is to record the probing depths for all teeth in any sextant scoring a 3 or 4 (using the CPITN score).*

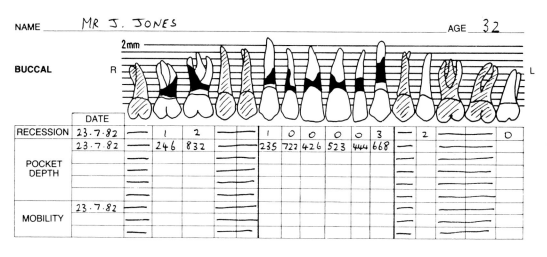

Fig. 5.9   *The final stage in recording probing depths is to shade in a pictorial representation of the probing depths. The horizontal lines can be used as a guide to aid in this – as the interval between each line represents 2 millimetres.*
Note that the recession is also recorded PICTORIALLY.

4. The probing depths are recorded, 6 measurements per tooth as in Fig. 5.8. Again for speed it is best to measure all the buccal depths (3 per tooth) for all teeth in each arch, then all the palatal or lingual depths.

5. Finally a pictorial representation can be drawn on the chart (Fig. 5.9). Although time-consuming, this is very useful on subsequent visits for dentist, hygienist and patient, because the areas that need attention can be immediately pinpointed at a glance. A mass of figures is usually meaningless to the patient and certainly more difficult for the dentist to interpret later.

Interpretation

Until recently the interpretation of pocket depths appeared to be a relatively simple procedure. Any pockets of 4mm or more were eliminated, usually using a surgical procedure. But over the last decade there has been increasing evidence to suggest that the apparent depth of the pocket and the true depth may not be the same.

The use of surgical techniques to eliminate pockets has also been questioned, as has the necessity for reducing probing depths at all in the absence of progressive disease. A recent paper by Badersten (3) even suggests that following scaling, root-planing and curettage it is necessary to wait at least 9 months (3) to establish the final result of the procedures on probing depths. This topic will be covered more fully in Chapter 11.

Where does this leave the general practitioner? Despite the lack of agreement on when to intervene surgically there is no doubt now that a knowledge of the periodontal condition is vital for control. Although measurement of probing depths has limitations it still provides a picture of the existing clinical situation with regard to loss of periodontal attachment, together with an indication of the destruction that has occurred in the past. If this information is combined with plaque and bleeding measurements (as described in the two previous chapters) then the practitioner is better able to understand how best to treat the individual patient.

Summary

Probing depths still remain the major periodontal index in the eyes of the profession and the administrators. Whilst there is some doubt as to the value of probing depths, until a better method of assessment is developed it seems likely that their use will continue to be best for monitoring the progression of disease. When deciding upon the necessity for surgical intervention probing depths must be known. In the presence of deepening probing depths, bleeding and good plaque control, surgery may well be indicated. This is covered in more detail in Chapter 11.

References

1. van der Velden, U. (1979): Probing force and the relationship of the probe tip to the periodontal tissues. Journal of Clinical Periodontology 6, 106-114.
2. Tromp J. A. H., Corba N. H. C., Borsboom P. C. F. & Fidler V. J. (1979): Reproducibility of a new pocket probe applying a constant force. Journal of Dental Research 58 2258. (Abstract)
3. Badersten A., Nilveus R. & Egelberg J., (1985): Effect of non-surgical periodontal therapy. VII Bleeding, suppuration and probing depth in sites with probing attachment loss. Journal of Clinical Periodontology 12. 432-440.

Chapter 6

Mobility and Overall Destruction

So far the periodontal indices we have described are relatively easy to collect. The presence or absence of plaque or bleeding, the depth of a pocket, or the identification of calculus are factors which can be assessed with little room for argument. But in the assessment of the mobility of a tooth, or the degree of overall periodontal destruction there is more room for differing interpretations. In this chapter we will discuss a mobility index and one assessment of overall destruction that we have found to be remarkably helpful clinically, despite its apparent complexity and the fact it was developed purely for epidemiological purposes. We will also mention our interpretation of the role of occlusion in periodontal disease, but hasten to point out that the oversimplified view we will give is merely a background to discussion of the mobility index and the interested reader is recommended to pursue this topic elsewhere.

The Role of the Occlusion

When considering the subject of occlusion one of the first obstacles that many dental practitioners perceive is their ability to measure mobility. How loose is loose? How important is mobility? What criteria are used in its measurement?

A second cause for concern amongst practitioners is the recent evidence suggesting that the only time mobility requires treatment (other than patient discomfort) is when that mobility can be shown to be progressively *increasing*. Within the clinical environment it can seem "wrong" to ignore a loose tooth simply because it is loose, although this is the way opinion is moving today. Despite this there is still a feeling amongst both patients and dentists that any mobile tooth should be treated.

Finally the importance of occlusal factors in periodontal therapy has been a much confused topic over the last decade. Is the occlusion to be considered in periodontal therapy? Should any occlusal factor be ignored? How important is obvious occlusal stress when preparing a treatment plan? These questions and more have caused the caring practitioner much concern because of apparently conflicting advice to be found in the literature.

Recent evidence suggests that occlusal forces play no part in the initiation of periodontal destruction, nor over reasonably long periods of time do they influence the rate of conversion of a gingivitis into a periodontitis. However in the presence of plaque there is some evidence to suggest that occlusal forces may cause a more rapid deterioration of an existing periodontitis (1).

The main finding, however, seems to be that even in the presence of occlusal disharmony, fastidious removal of supra and subgingival plaque *alone* will prevent further *periodontal* destruction, given that the point of periodontal tissue loss has not become so great that a traumatic luxation might occur. This emphasises the importance of plaque control and scaling as the elements with the greatest priority in situations where occlusal disorders and periodontal disease exist side by side. This conclusion removes the necessity for the general practitioner to worry about correcting occlusal disharmonies as the treatment of first choice, and allows time for periodontal healing to occur following traditional therapy.

We feel it is important to restate this approach. In the presence of inflammatory disease and occlusal disharmony the emphasis should be more on the correction of the inflammatory component of disease by the traditional methods of plaque control and scaling with monitoring to evaluate the results. Only when the inflammatory disease is under control is it appropriate to investigate the occlusion and to consider treatment of any disharmony by the appropriate means.

However, in the presence of symptoms from occlusal disharmony (muscle spasm, severe bruxism and wear, pain in the temporomandibular joints, etc.) there is obviously a need for occlusal investigation as well as for traditional periodontal therapy. The important point is that such an investigation is not for periodontal reasons but to help the occlusal symptoms.

Measurement of Mobility

Mobility is recorded using the index in Fig. 6.1. It is usually estimated by moving the tooth with the tip of a probe in a fissure or placing the handle of an instrument and a finger on opposite sides of the tooth. The tooth is moved laterally and the degree of movement assessed against the table (Fig. 6.1). The appropriate score is then recorded on the Probing Depth Chart (Fig. 6.2).

Because of the evidence that it is *increasing* mobility which is significant (2) it becomes important to record an

GRADE 0
No apparent mobility.

GRADE 1
Perceptible mobility but
less than 1 mm buccolingually.

GRADE 2
Definite mobility
between 1-2 mm.

GRADE 3
Gross mobility
exceeding 2 mm buccolingually
and/or vertical mobility.

Fig. 6.1   Mobility Index Scores

PROBING DEPTH CHART

NAME   MR S. BROWN

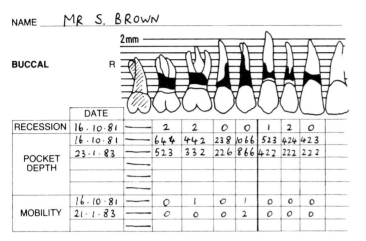

BUCCAL

	DATE								
RECESSION	16.10.81	—	2	2	0	0	1	2	0
POCKET DEPTH	16.10.81	—	644	442	238	066	523	424	423
	23.1.83	—	523	332	226	866	422	222	222
		—							
		—							
MOBILITY	16.10.81	—	0	1	0	1	0	0	0
	21.1.83	—	0	0	0	2	0	0	0

Fig. 6.2 In this figure the upper right first premolar (14) and first molar (16) both had a mobility score of 1 on initial examination. On re-examination 15 months later the score for the molar is zero but for the premolar it has increased to two – signifying a deterioration.

estimate of the degree of mobility on initial and subsequent visits, as seen in Fig. 6.2.

This records the situation of the upper right first premolar which had deep pocketing on the initial visit in 1981. In 1983 the mobility had increased although the pocketing had reduced slightly in depth. This was a situation in which some treatment was required.

Interpretation of Mobility

As mentioned above the low grades of mobility often seen at an initial visit need not be a cause for concern. Looseness alone is not an indication for treatment and a surprisingly large number of patients are unaware of their loose teeth. In fact it is wise not to emphasise mobility scores where treatment is not indicated because the patient may start to exhibit unnecessary anxiety once the mobility is drawn to their attention.

One of the clinical mistakes of the past was the splinting of all loose teeth to remove mobility for its own sake. Unless this mobility is a concern of the patient (which is rare) it is much better to note the mobility score and leave the tooth alone (in the absence of occlusal symptoms). Splinting should be contemplated only if the mobility is increasing or if the patient finds the looseness uncomfortable. Even then occlusal adjustment rather than some type of splinting is a preferable technique as it will decrease the forces on the tooth and hence probably reduce the mobility without the placement of a plaque-trapping appliance such as a splint.

Measurement of Overall Periodontal Destruction (Periodontal Index)

Knowledge of the overall periodontal destruction together with the patient's age gives an idea of prognosis. In 1956 Russell produced an index of periodontal destruction (PI) for epidemiological purposes (2), and although this index can be heavily criticised as being irrelevant to general practice, in our hands it has been found to be accurate, representative, easy to measure and suitable for interpretation.

Measuring the P.I.

This index is not an easy one to understand at first glance although it is extremely simple to record in everyday practice providing that the other indices (probing depths, bleeding, etc.) have been recorded first.

The parameters for the index are listed in Fig. 6.3.

In reality this index can be simplified as follows:

Any tooth with a pocket of 4 mm or over is Grade 6 (unless Grade 8 which is rarely scored).

All other teeth will be Grade 2 (inflammation around the entire tooth), Grade 1 (inflammation around half the tooth) or Grade 0 (no inflammation at all).

Thus if the Periodontal Index is taken *after* probing depths have been measured and mobility assessed the D.S.A. can determine how many teeth are Grade 6 by consulting the probing depth. She will immediately see which

---

GRADE 0
NEGATIVE — no overt inflamation in the investing tissues nor loss of function due to destruction of the supporting tissues.

GRADE 1
MILD GINGIVITIS — overt inflammation in the free gingivae which does not circumscribe the tooth.

GRADE 2
GINGIVITIS — inflammation completely circumscribing the tooth but no break in the epithelial attachment.

GRADE 6
GINGIVITIS WITH POCKET FORMATION — the epithelial attachment has been broken and there is a pocket (not merely a deepened gingival crevice due to swelling in the free gingivae). There is no interference with normal masticatory function, the tooth is firm in its socket and has not drifted.

GRADE 8
ADVANCED DESTRUCTION WITH LOSS OF MASTICATORY FUNCTION — the tooth may be loose, may have drifted, may sound dull on percussion with a metallic instrument, may be depressible in its socket.

Fig. 6.3 Russell's Periodontal Index Scores

teeth have probing depths of 4 mm or more and can note these measurements (Fig. 6.4) without any necessity for the dentist to look at them.

It now becomes a simple matter for the D.S.A. to call out the remaining teeth and for the dentist to assess each tooth clinically as a 0, 1 or 2. These are then recorded on a chart as in Fig. 6.5. Finally the figures are totalled and the

PERIODONTAL INDEX

		6	6	6	6				6		6	6			6	
8	7	6	5	4	3	2	1	1	2	3	4	5	6	7	8
8	7	6	5	4	3	2	1	1	2	3	4	5	6	7	8
		6	6	6		6								6		

TOTAL SCORE / NUMBER OF TEETH = ▢

TOTAL SCORE / NUMBER OF TEETH = ▢

Fig. 6.4   When calculating the P.I. the first stage is to record the teeth with probing depths of 4 millimetres or more (using the probing depth chart scores). These teeth are given a score of 6. Occasionally a score of 8 may be more accurate as in the case of gross mobility.

PERIODONTAL INDEX

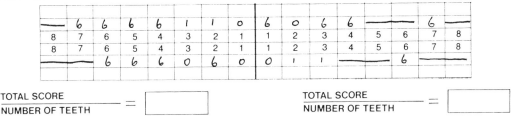

		6	6	6	6	1	1	0	6	0	6	6			6	
8	7	6	5	4	3	2	1	1	2	3	4	5	6	7	8
8	7	6	5	4	3	2	1	1	2	3	4	5	6	7	8
		6	6	6	0	6	0	0	1	1			6			

TOTAL SCORE / NUMBER OF TEETH = ▢

TOTAL SCORE / NUMBER OF TEETH = ▢

Fig. 6.5   The next stage when calculating the P.I. is to estimate the scores of the remaining teeth as 2 (inflammation fully around the tooth), or 1 (inflammation around approximately half the tooth), or zero (no inflammation). This is done clinically.

PERIODONTAL INDEX

		6	6	6	6	1	1	0	6	0	6	6			6	
8	7	6	5	4	3	2	1	1	2	3	4	5	6	7	8
8	7	6	5	4	3	2	1	1	2	3	4	5	6	7	8
		6	6	6	0	6	0	0	1	1			6			

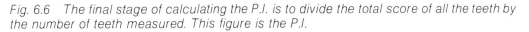

TOTAL SCORE 82 / NUMBER OF TEETH 22 = 3 · 73

TOTAL SCORE / NUMBER OF TEETH = ▢

Fig. 6.6   The final stage of calculating the P.I. is to divide the total score of all the teeth by the number of teeth measured. This figure is the P.I.

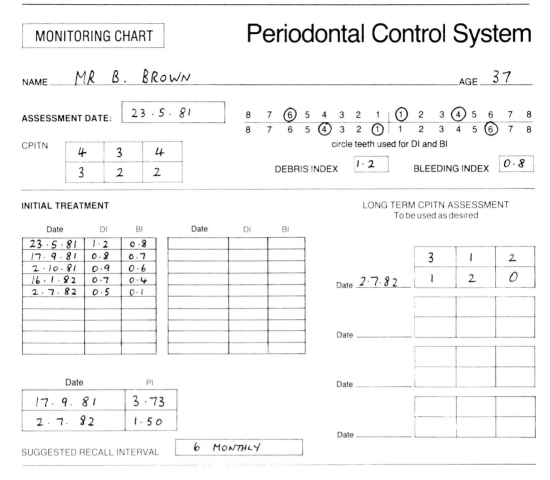

MONITORING CHART

Periodontal Control System

NAME MR B. BROWN   AGE 37

ASSESSMENT DATE: 23 . 5 . 81

8	7	⑥	5	4	3	2	1	①	2	3	④	5	6	7	8
8	7	6	5	④	3	2	①	1	2	3	4	5	⑥	7	8

circle teeth used for DI and BI

CPITN

4	3	4
3	2	2

DEBRIS INDEX 1·2   BLEEDING INDEX 0·8

INITIAL TREATMENT

Date	DI	BI
23 · 5 · 81	1·2	0·8
17 · 9 · 81	0·8	0·7
2 · 10 · 81	0·9	0·6
16 · 1 · 82	0·7	0·4
2 · 7 · 82	0·5	0·1

Date	DI	BI

Date	PI
17 · 9 · 81	3 · 73
2 · 7 · 82	1 · 50

SUGGESTED RECALL INTERVAL   6 MONTHLY

LONG TERM CPITN ASSESSMENT
To be used as desired

Date 2·7·82

3	1	2
1	2	0

Date _____

Date _____

Date _____

Date _____

Fig. 6.7   *The Monitoring Chart is used as an overall chart for the patient's periodontal health. On first visit in May 1981 the patient is assessed using the CPITN, D.I. and B.I. as in the upper portion of the chart.*
If further treatment is required then in the initial stages (which can last several years in certain cases) the D.I. and B.I. are taken at the start of every visit for periodontal care and the results recorded. In this case there has been a steady improvement in both plaque control and gingival health.
The patient is assessed as being under control in July 1982 and the P.I. retaken. This shows an improvement from 3.87 to 1.50. At the same time the CPITN is retaken, also showing an improvement. From the total assessment the dentist decides to recommend 6-monthly visits for recall maintenance.

resultant figure divided by the number of teeth to obtain an average score — which becomes the Periodontal Index (Fig. 6.6).

This figure is then recorded on the Monitoring Chart and later after treatment the adjusted figure can also be recorded as in Fig. 6.7.

Assessment of the Periodontal Index

When measuring the Periodontal Index several difficulties can arise for the inexperienced operator. One of these has already been mentioned in Chapter 4 — the difficulty of assessing the degree of inflammation. From a practical point of view it would seem sensible to include florid inflammation in the scores 1 or 2 (so that mild bleeding on probing without any other obvious indication of inflammation would score a 0). Scores of 8 are assigned only when the teeth involved are virtually requiring extraction.

In the use of the PI it is important that each operator selects his or her own judgemental criteria and continues to use them in the longitudinal monitoring of patients. If this is done then difficulties in interpretation should not occur.

Summary

Mobility and overall destruction indices are two that appear more susceptible to difficulties in scoring and interpretation than most. However once the practitioner or hygienist has gained initial experience in recording these indices they should find that familiarity creates confidence, and the extra information obtained from adding the Mobility Index and the Periodontal Index to the repertoire of diagnostic criteria is well worth the little additional time they require.

References

1. Lindhe J. & Svanberg G. (1974): Influence of trauma from occlusion on progression of experimental periodontitis in the Beagle dog. Journal of Clinical Periodontology 1 3-14.

2. Russell A. L., (1956): A system of classification and scoring for prevalence surveys of periodontal disease. Journal of Dental Research 35 350-359.

TREATMENT OF PATIENTS

In Chapter 1 we mentioned the importance of finding a structure which would allow the patient, dentist, hygienist and any remunerating authority to respond to the concept of "continuing care". We suggested that monitoring provided just such a structure, and in Part 2 we have identified a variety of different indices which are required to create that structure in practice.

The use of these indices in the identification and treatment of patients forms the content of Part 3 of this book. We have taken the step of using a system of categorisation of patients, ranging from A to E with A referring to the patients with the least amount of treatment required and E referring to patients who require substantial care.

Thus Category A patients require only very simple periodontal treatment involving removal of subgingival calculus and oral hygiene instruction. Category B patients require more extensive treatment but have no loss of attachment and pocketing, whilst Category C patients have bleeding and pockets not exceeding 5mm in depth. Category D patients have fairly extensive disease with pockets exceeding 5mm but respond well to treatment, whilst Category E patients are those who are very susceptible to the disease process and do not respond well to traditional therapy.

We are aware that there will be some patients who fall on the dividing lines within this simplified classification system, but it is our belief that such a system facilitates interpretation of the indices and subsequent planning of treatment. Furthermore the age factor must be taken into account, because if there are both young and old patients in a given category the younger patients will have a worse prognosis. With these limitations in mind we can begin to categorise our patients by the methods described in the following section of the book. The types of diagnoses and eventual treatment needed by each group will then be apparent.

Chapter 7

Selecting Patients for Periodontal Treatment

This chapter considers the selection of patients in a dental practice for collection of indices. Furthermore the important question — "can some of the indices be omitted for some of the patients who qualify for selection?" will be discussed. As mentioned in the introduction to Part 3 we have created categories for patients suffering from periodontal disease, but it should be noted at once that even for patients with no obvious periodontal disease some measurements are useful in providing baseline data against which changes in the future might be compared.

Initial Selection

The identification of patients who need to have periodontal indices recorded is still controversial and open to different interpretation by different authorities. Certain studies would suggest that 99% of the population have some periodontal disease and therefore require treatment (1). Nevertheless, as most dentists are aware, many of their patients can tolerate higher plaque levels and even limited gingival inflammation without immediate harm or progression of disease.

A point arises from the personal experience of one of us in general dental practice and has been corroborated since by many other dentists. It is simply that much periodontal disease can continue unnoticed by even the most caring practitioner in a busy practice when a routine method of periodontal probing is not carried out for every patient.

The answer to the question — "Which patients require a form of monitoring?" — falls somewhere between two diametrically opposite approaches to treatment. One states that virtually every patient must be regarded as requiring continuing periodontal care. The other view assumes that in most patients the disease will probably not progress seriously within their expected lifetime, thus monitoring would be regarded as overtreatment.

It would seem to us that the confict is most easily resolved by recommending the use of a simple index for the routine collection of data on all patients, and if this shows certain levels of disease then further investigation should follow. The CPITN and its associated probe mentioned in Chapter 2 are ideal for this purpose.

Patient Categories

The following system of patient classification provides a simplified means of categorising patients into groups requiring different treatment and different indices in monitoring.

CATEGORY A: Patients who appear to be resistant to periodontal disease and who require only simple scaling and ocasional plaque control instruction.

CATEGORY B: Patients who require regular visits for scaling in selected areas together with plaque control instruction — often because of the amount of calculus they form. These patients may have a few shallow pockets of up to 4 mm but usually have little loss of attachment and pocketing.

CATEGORY C: Patients with early destructive disease but with pockets not exceeding 6 mm in any one sextant.

CATEGORY D: Patients with more extensive signs of periodontal disease, including some deep pocketing of over 6 mm, bleeding, bone loss, mobility and even pus formation. These patients respond to therapy and can be controlled fairly easily.

CATEGORY E: Patients with a heightened susceptibility to periodontal disease who tend to continue to deteriorate despite good plaque control and extensive therapy.

Although these categories are somewhat artificial they can form the backbone of a sensitive agreement between dentist, hygienist and patient and where appropriate can help the dentist to apply for prior approval to treat from either an insurance scheme or a State controlled system of health care.

Using the CPITN

This index was originally devised for epidemiological purposes but has been adapted for use in general practice (2) as described in Chapter 2. What is needed is an extension of the present grading system (see Chapter 2) to help in categorising patients into groups A, B, C, D or E and thereby to allow the dentist to identify further indices and when necessary radiographs which will help in monitoring these patients in the future.

CPITN SCORES: Mainly 0 and 1, or possibly 2 in lower anterior or upper molar regions only.
Category A
Suggested indices: D.I. and B.I.

CPITN SCORES: 2 in upper anterior and lower posterior regions.
Category B
Suggested indices: D.I. and B.I.

CPITN SCORES: 3 anywhere in the mouth.
Category C
Suggested indices: D.I., B.I., Bleeding Points Chart, and Probing Depths Chart.

CPITN SCORES: 4 or * anywhere in the mouth.
Categories D and E
Suggested indices: B.I., D.I., Bleeding Points Chart, Probing Depth Chart, Mobility Index and Periodontal Index.

It should be noted that Category E patients will only be apparent after they have failed to respond to treatment.

Indications of Radiographs

For Category C patients bitewing or panoramic radiographs should be taken in case of bone loss.

For Category D or E patients individual intraoral radiographs are necessary for teeth showing furcation involvements or total loss of attachment of more than 7 mms.

It should be noted that Patients in Categories D or E cannot be distinguished at this stage as they are only identified by the eventual response to treatment.

EXAMPLES

Patient 1.

3	1	2
2	2	2

CATEGORY: C

Suggested indices: DI and BI probing depth chart upper right sextant.

Comments: Although this patient has only one sextant with pockets over 3.5 mm in depth it is important to prepare a probing depth chart of that sextant to identify those areas. At its simplest this will mean probing depth measurements of four teeth upon completion of the oral hygiene instruction (scaling) and polishing of the sextants scoring 3. However, some dentists may regard it as important to be aware of the probing depths in other areas in case a deterioration should occur in the future. This can be determined only if the original probing depths were known.

As an additional safeguard, bitewing radiographs to show undetected bone loss should be taken of sextants scoring 3.

Finally, it is likely that such patients should be seen for recalls at six-monthly intervals.

Patient 2.

2	0	1
1	2	1

CATEGORY: A

Suggested indices: D.I and B.I.

Comments: the presence of calculus in the lower anterior region and right posterior molar region is consistent with the formation of supragingival calculus in these areas and probably requires very little attention. The Bleeding Index and Debris Index are required purely to provide base-line data should the situation deteriorate. There is less concern about a recall period for such patients than for those with sextants scoring 3 or more. Nevertheless recall for scaling should be considered at least once a year.

EXAMPLES

Patient 3.

4	3	4
4	2	2

CATEGORY: D

Suggested indices: all indices.

Comments: This patient has advanced pocketing in three sextants and is almost certainly highly susceptible to periodontal disease. If future treatment fails to create a definite improvement this patient will move into Category E.

It is possible that following careful scaling and root planing (possibly with surgery later) this patient would respond so well to therapy that he or she would move into Category B — this would become apparent only on future monitoring using all the indices.

This patient may well be referred to a specialist periodontist for treatment and subsequently monitored by the practitioner to ensure that should an active phase of disease develop again the patient can be referred back for further treatment.

Patient 4

2	2	2
2	2	2

CATEGORY: B

Suggested indices: D.I. and B.I.

Comments: this patient would require fairly extensive plaque control instruction and scaling to remove the hard deposits, but the lack of pocketing in any sextant suggests a patient who is resistant to periodontal disease. What is not known is the degree of loss of attachment (due to the limitation of the CPITN) and in some cases this patient might be classified as a Category C due to recession and generalised loss of periodontal support.

Such a patient highlights the importance of a complete diagnosis and the limitations of attempting to use periodontal indices alone, without additional supporting clinical data.

Interpretation

Although the majority of cases will fall neatly into one category or another there will be certain patients who fall into the "grey" areas between. An example is the patient with very little disease present and minimal calculus who when examined has a single pocket of 4 mm around an upper molar.

By the same token a patient with no pocketing and only 4 scores of 2 in the posterior sextants could require extensive scaling (especially subgingivally) taking several visits to complete.

Despite these exceptions the majority of patients will fall into the categories described and the recommended treatment would be as described.

This is summarised in Fig. 7.

The Use of Radiographs

Routine bitewing radiographic examination can help in the diagnosis and monitoring of the disease, the identification of early bone loss, disclosing the presence of subgingival calculus and angular bone resorption. Unless a standardised technique is used routinely, long term radiographic monitoring should be approached with caution, as varying tube angulation can result in differing appearances on the radiograph. One situation in which radiographs can be particularly useful is in the identification of previously active zones with pocket formation which may not now be apparent clinically. The periodontal probe should not penetrate a long epithelial attachment if the correct pressure is used and thus an area of potentially rapid breakdown during a future active cycle of the disease could be missed. For this reason initial radiographs to show the condition of interdental bone in sextants with a CPITN score of 3 or more are recommended.

Summary

Patient selection for periodontal therapy is one of the most difficult aspects of the provision of care. Although open to some degree of interpretation in individual cases a quantifiable method of assessment such as the CPITN provides would seem to have advantages for both the dentist and the agency meeting treatment costs.

By extending the grading system of the CPITN to allow categorisation of individual patients it becomes possible to simplify the selection of indices to be used and the treatment to be applied.

References

1. Sheiham A. (1969): The prevalence and severity of periodontal disease in British populations. British Dental Journal 126 115-122.
2. Croxson L.J. (1984): A simplified periodontal screening examination: the Community Periodontal Index of Treatment Needs (WHO) in general practice. International Dental Journal 34 28-34.

Category	Clinical description	CPITN Scores	Suggested Indices	Recommended treatment	Follow-up
A	Mainly healthy, but bleeding on probing, supragingival deposits of calculus in the lower anteriors and buccal to upper molars	0, 1 and possibly 2 in lower anterior or upper posterior region	Debris Index Bleeding Index	Selected scaling and O.H.I.	6 months
B	Large amounts of calculus or profuse gingival bleeding. No pockets of over 3.5 mm	2 in lower molar and upper anterior regions	Debris Index Bleeding Index	Extensive scaling of the areas that need it. O.H.I.	6 months
C	Periodontal destruction comprising a few pockets of 5 mm or less, some bleeding and calculus	3 in one or more segments	Debris Index Bleeding Index Bleeding Points	Scaling and O.H.I. Root planing and subgingival curettage if applicable	6 months
D	Any periodontal destruction, from a few pockets, bleeding and calculus to deep active pocketing, mobility and pus formation. Also other types of infection such as A.U.G.	4 or * and high D.I.	Debris Index Bleeding Index Probing depths in some cases Bleeding points Mobility	Scaling and O.H.I. Root planing and subgingival curettage where applicable. Possibly surgery later	Maybe 3 months or possibly 6
E	Heightened suscepti- bility to periodontal disease despite treatment and good plaque control. The same signs as Category D	4 or * but low D.I.	Debris Index Bleeding Index Probing Depths Bleeding points Mobility	Scaling and O.H.I. Root planing and subgingival curettage where applicable. Possibly surgery later	Essential for 2 or 3 months

Figure 7.1   *Suggested Treatment linked to CPITN Gradings.*

Chapter 8

Treating Category A and B Patients

So far in Part 3 we have discussed the different categories that can be used to help select patients and stated that the CPITN can play a helpful role in this selection. A brief description of which indices besides CPITN can help in both diagnosis, treatment and follow-up was given in Fig. 7.3. The next 3 chapters enlarge on this and give suggested applications for the other indices mentioned in Part 2.

This chapter is concerned with patients who fall into Categories A and B. Most will require only the Debris and Bleeding Indices (D.I. and B.I.), a point of importance when considerations of time have to be taken into account.

Distinguishing Category A and B Patients

As we have seen in the last chapter patients placed in Category A or B at the initial visit will be patients with virtually no periodontal pocketing but with varying degrees of gingival inflammation and calculus. We consider that the patient will be in Category B rather than Category A if he or she has calculus on teeth other than the lower anteriors or upper molars (as these areas are usually the sites where supragingival calculus forms in patients with an otherwise healthy mouth).

Obviously this classification cannot be all-embracing. Certain patients will have an over-reaction to plaque resulting in excessive gingival bleeding but with very little calculus, thus qualifying for Category B. Others may have small insignificant deposits of supragingival calculus in the upper anterior region which, by the strict definition would place them in Category B, but commonsense suggests they should be classified as Category A only. Similarly patients without pocketing may have extensive gingival recession and the subsequent loss of attachment would qualify them for Category D (requiring more extensive therapy). A similar situation can arise if furcation involvement is detected.

Although these situations are uncommon, they are possible and consequently other periodontal indices are required to clarify a situation initially revealed by the CPITN alone. Fortunately though, in the majority of patients the simple classification described in the last chapter (Fig. 7.3) is sufficient for their categorisation.

Refining the Picture

In photography a simple picture can appear blurred, when with better focussing a clearer image would have been obtained. In the same way the clinical situation suggested by the CPITN will be clarified by the use of the Debris Index and the Bleeding Index.

As already discussed in Chapters 3 and 4 for the following reasons both indices have been selected to form the back-bone of the Periodontal Control System.

- they are not time-consuming to record.
- they reflect changes in plaque control and inflammation very quickly.
- dentist and hygienist can calibrate themselves easily.
- they can be readily interpreted by patients and they aid in the provision of information.
- they aid in patient motivation.
- they can indicate a sudden change in inflammation (which may be an indicator of a burst of disease) which can be related to the plaque levels at the same time.
- they can be understood by clerical staff administering payment.

Because the element of time plays such an important role in interpretation of disease patterns it is helpful to have a record of the D.I. and B.I. *prior* to a burst of activity, and thus we recommend that both indices are routinely scored when-ever visits are made for periodontal assessment or treatment. This can mean that the dentist or hygienist may be recording zero scores in apparently healthy mouths which could be con-strued as "wasting time". As the dis-cussion which now follows will show, nothing could be further from the truth. Fig. 8.1 shows that if time is spent taking the D.I. and B.I. routinely then should a

burst of activity occur or the patient's oral hygiene lapse (for whatever reason) it would be easier to obtain approval from either the patient or other interested party for a more comprehensive course of periodontal therapy than if records did not exist. The chart in Fig. 8.1 clearly shows a sudden increase in the B.I. (from levels of 0 to 0.8) yet the D.I. is still very low (0.5). One interpretation of the

LONG TERM TREATMENT

Date	DI	BI
16.5.79	0.5	0.2
23.7.80	0.7	0.1
6.2.81	0.4	0
2.8.81	0.5	0
7.3.82	0.2	0.3
20.10.82	0.5	0
16.6.83	0.3	0.2
8.3.84	0.7	0.1
13.10.84	0.4	0.3
12.8.85	0.3	0
16.6.86	0.5	0.8
21.12.86	0.2	0.3

Fig. 8.1 By comparing the D.I. and B.I. scores over the period a guide of the trend of plaque control and gingival health becomes apparent. Note the sudden increase in bleeding (B.I. = 0.8) in June 1986 without a corres-ponding increase in plaque score. This is a danger sign that perhaps a "burst" of disease activity is happening. The dentist's response is to see the patient after only 6 months whereas the recall intervals had been stretching to 9 and 10 months prior to this event.

figures is that despite a continuing high standard of plaque control there is an increase in gingival response, causing bleeding, which *could* be a prelude to a burst of disease.

A second bonus derived from collecting indices prior to their obvious need is that, following such a "burst", it is easy to demonstrate to the patient that treatment is necessary. This facilitates discussion with the patient over its cost.

Recording the Indices

In order to ensure that the D.I. and B.I. are recorded properly a systematic method of recording the figures is essential. Various charts, forms and grids have been devised by different operators in the past and all have their merits. Our attempts to devise a simple system which is both comprehensive and useful for longterm assessment has

led us to the MONITORING CHART and INDEX CALCULATOR seen in Figs. 8.3 and 8.4 (overleaf).

The method of scoring the D.I. and B.I. was described in Chapters 3 and 4 and the individual scores for the 6 selected Ramfjord teeth recorded on the Index Calculator as in Fig. 8.2.a.

To understand this more fully consider the 4 scores for the upper right molar (Fig. 8.2.b). The D.I. scores of 1 for the buccal surface and 2 for the palatal surface, mean that more than one third (but less than two thirds) of the palatal surface of the molar is covered with plaque whilst there is less than one third coverage on the buccal surface. The score of 1 *could* also mean that whilst running the probe gently within the sulcus buccally to check for bleeding a fine line of sulcular plaque was detected even though none was visible after disclosing.

TOOTH	SURFACE	DI	BI	DI	B
6⌋ (16)	buccal	1	0		
	lingual	2	1		
⌊1 (21)	buccal	0	0		
	lingual	0	0		
⌊4 (24)	buccal	1	1		
	lingual	1	2		
⌈6 (36)	buccal	1	0		
	lingual	2	2		
7⌉ (41)	buccal	2	2		
	lingual	3	2		
4⌉ (44)	buccal	0	0		
	lingual	3	1		
TOTAL SCORE		16	11		
INDEX		1·3	0·9		

DI	BI	DI
1	0	
2	1	

Fig. 8.2 (b)   This section of the Index Calculator is used simply to note down the scores, making the actual calculation of the D.I. and B.I. simpler.

Fig. 8.2 (a)   The Index Calculator Form.

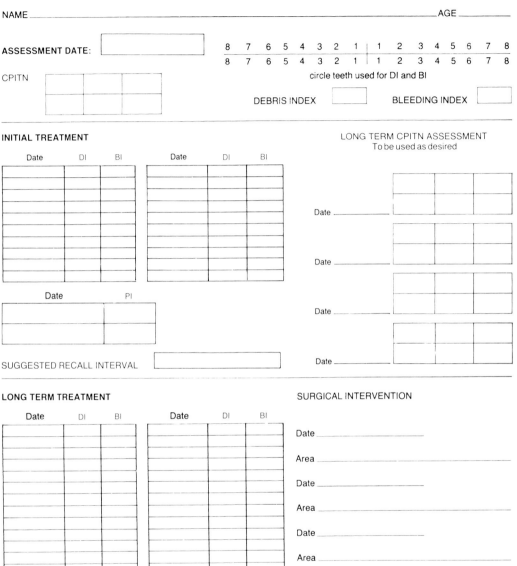

MONITORING CHART

Periodontal Control System

NAME_____AGE_____

ASSESSMENT DATE:

| 8 | 7 | 6 | 5 | 4 | 3 | 2 | 1 | | 1 | 2 | 3 | 4 | 5 | 6 | 7 | 8 |
| 8 | 7 | 6 | 5 | 4 | 3 | 2 | 1 | | 1 | 2 | 3 | 4 | 5 | 6 | 7 | 8 |

circle teeth used for DI and BI

CPITN

DEBRIS INDEX   BLEEDING INDEX

INITIAL TREATMENT

| Date | DI | BI |
| Date | DI | BI |

| Date | PI |

SUGGESTED RECALL INTERVAL

LONG TERM CPITN ASSESSMENT
To be used as desired

Date _____

Date _____

Date _____

Date _____

Date _____

LONG TERM TREATMENT

| Date | DI | BI |
| Date | DI | BI |

SURGICAL INTERVENTION

Date _____

Area _____

Date _____

Area _____

Date _____

Area _____

Date _____

Area _____

Date _____

Area _____

Date _____

Area _____

Date _____

Area _____

70   *Fig. 8.3   The Monitoring Chart*

Periodontal Control System

NAME _____

PERIODONTAL INDEX

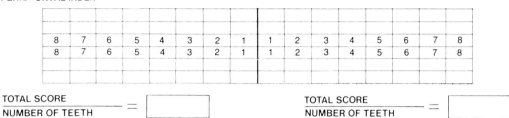

8	7	6	5	4	3	2	1	1	2	3	4	5	6	7	8
8	7	6	5	4	3	2	1	1	2	3	4	5	6	7	8

$$\frac{\text{TOTAL SCORE}}{\text{NUMBER OF TEETH}} = \boxed{}$$

$$\frac{\text{TOTAL SCORE}}{\text{NUMBER OF TEETH}} = \boxed{}$$

DI & BI SCORES

TOOTH	SURFACE	SCORE													
		DI	BI	DI	BI	DI	BI	DI	BI	DI	BI	DI	BI	DI	BI
	buccal														
	lingual														
	buccal														
	lingual														
	buccal														
	lingual														
	buccal														
	lingual														
	buccal														
	lingual														
	buccal														
	lingual														
TOTAL SCORE															
INDEX															

TOOTH	SURFACE	SCORE													
		DI	BI	DI	BI	DI	BI	DI	BI	DI	BI	DI	BI	DI	BI
	buccal														
	lingual														
	buccal														
	lingual														
	buccal														
	lingual														
	buccal														
	lingual														
	buccal														
	lingual														
	buccal														
	lingual														
TOTAL SCORE															
INDEX															

Fig. 8.4   The Index Calculator.

The B.I. scores of 0 buccally and 1 palatally indicate that there was no bleeding buccally and delayed bleeding on the palatal surface after running the probe in the sulcus.

We have found that if the dentist calls out the two D.I. scores followed by the two B.I. scores for each tooth in turn, the D.S.A. can record the 4 figures as in Fig. 8.2.b.

If the scores are now totalled (in the boxes below) and then averaged (divided by 12 in this case) the index can be calculated. The next step is to circle the selected teeth on the Monitoring Chart as in Fig. 8.5. This is to ensure that the same teeth are measured at subsequent visits by the dentist or hygienist.

Thus the Monitoring Chart enables the *trend* of the D.I. and B.I. to be seen over a long period of continuing periodontal care. It will show fluctuations in both patient behaviour (oral hygiene) and the response of the periodontium (gingival inflammation).

The Concept of Trend

This concept of a *trend* in the figures is a vital one within the Periodontal Control System, for it demonstrates the real value of the system. A single recording of the D.I. has only limited use, rather like a snapshot of the oral hygiene at any one moment. But following the history of the patient's oral hygiene over several years

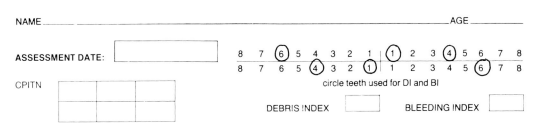

Fig. 8.5

Finally the scores for the D.I. and B.I. are recorded with the date on the Monitoring Chart. The reason for transferring the indices across to the Monitoring Chart is to enable the dentist and patient to see a very clear picture emerging with the passage of time. Fig. 8.6 compares several recordings of both indices over several years and demonstrates this point very well.

will reveal change that may occur due to external circumstances. This may be a dramatic event such as the illness of a spouse or problems at home, or just to a lack of communication on the part of the dentist.

If the change is slight it may well go unnoticed because of the small difference in plaque control at each recall visit, but will be noticeable in the record provided by the Periodontal Control System. Fig. 8.7 (overleaf) shows just such a trend which will be identified by the dentist or hygienist who can then take the appropriate steps to elicit the cause.

After an initial improvement in the D.I. (from 0.8 to 0.5 over a 2 year period) and a corresponding improvement in the B.I. there has been a steady rise in the D.I. (beyond 1.0 which is worse than seen on first examination). The B.I. is still reason-able (0.6 is unlikely to cause any worry-ing symptoms to the patient) thus not alerting either patient or practitioner.

It is unlikely that such a small and slow change would have been picked up by the same dentist over a period of time, and even if the disease remained stable, despite the higher levels of plaque, a sudden burst of active disease could have caused a more serious deteriora-tion than if the level of plaque had been kept under control.

Summary

There is no doubt that although the CPITN gives a good overall picture of the clinical situation and need for treatment, it is somewhat limited when used as the sole index. A particular limitation is the measurement of changes in the patient as a response to therapy over a short period of time. There are also some situa-tions where use of the CPITN alone can

INITIAL TREATMENT

Date	DI	BI
17.5.82	1·3	0·9
23·7·82	1·0	0·9
6·1·83	0·6	0·4
14·7·83	0·75	0·5
2·2·84	0·25	0·3
3·7·84	0·4	0·17

Fig. 8.6   Part A

TOOTH	SURFACE	SCORE													
		DI	BI	DI	BI	DI	BI	DI	BI	DI	BI	DI	BI	DI	BI
6⌋ (16)	buccal	1	0	1	1	0	0	0	0	0	0	0	0		
	lingual	2	1	1	1	1	1	1	1	0	0	1	0		
L⌋ (21)	buccal	0	0	0	0	0	0	0	0	0	0	0	0		
	lingual	0	0	1	0	1	0	0	0	0	1	0	0		
⌊4 (24)	buccal	1	1	0	0	0	0	1	0	0	0	0	0		
	lingual	1	2	1	1	1	1	1	1	1	1	1	1		
⌈6 (36)	buccal	1	0	1	1	0	0	1	1	0	0	0	0		
	lingual	2	2	2	2	1	1	2	2	1	0	0	0		
⌐1 (41)	buccal	2	2	1	2	1	0	1	0	0	0	0	0		
	lingual	3	2	2	2	1	1	1	1	1	1	1	0		
4⌐ (44)	buccal	0	0	0	0	0	0	0	0	0	0	1	0		
	lingual	3	1	2	1	1	1	1	0	0	1	1	1		
TOTAL SCORE		16	11	12	11	7	5	9	6	3	4	5	2		
INDEX		1·3	0·9	1·0	0·9	0·6	0·4	0·75	0·5	0·25	0·3	0·4	0·17		

Fig. 8.6   Part B

Date	DI	BI
8.5.79	0.8	0.3
16.7.79	0.7	0.3
3.1.80	0.5	0.1
4.3.80	0.3	0
16.9.80	0.4	0
11.4.81	0.6	0.2
2.10.81	0.5	0
13.8.82	0.7	0.1
6.3.83	0.7	0.2
23.10.83	0.9	0.1
17.6.84	0.9	0.3
14.12.84	1.1	0.4
23.7.85	1.3	0.6
17.10.85	0.9	0.4
3.4.86	0.6	0.1
23.9.86	0.5	0
17.3.87	0.3	0

Fig. 8.7

be either inadequate or misleading when dealing with individuals.

By including other periodontal indices in the initial clinical assessment a much better appreciation of both the baseline situation and the reaction to therapy can be gained. When considering patients with gingival inflammation only, together with little or no loss of attachment (Categories A and B patients), the use of the Debris and Bleeding Indices alone is sufficient.

Although using these indices may seem at times to be recording the obvious the value will be seen after a burst of disease. Because active periodontal disease can be an intermittent yet rapidly evolving disease, past records become increasingly valuable in the assessment of prognosis and the planning for further treatment.

Chapter 9

Treating Category C, D and E Patients

The common feature distinguishing Category C, D and E patients from others is that they all have some degree of periodontal destruction with loss of attachment resulting in pocketing. There is tremendous variation however within these categories. The range is from the person who has just started to develop an isolated pocket around one tooth with the disease process confined to the gingiva elsewhere, to the patient with periodontal abscesses, pus, mobility, drifting of teeth and generalised pocketing throughout the mouth.

Category C patients among this group are easy to identify because no sextant scores more than Code 3 (CPITN). Furthermore, their treatment is simpler (similar to that for Category B patients mentioned in the last chapter) and revolves around simple monitoring, oral hygiene instruction and scaling. The main *difference* in approach for the dentist or hygienist between the category B and category C patient is the need to focus more diagnostic attention upon the sextants scoring 3. This usually requires the use of the probing chart *for the appropriate sextants only*, i.e. for those areas still scoring 3 following initial therapy. Another difference between the B and C patients is that the Category C patient may require more frequent recalls.

At an initial visit however it is almost impossible to distinguish between patients who will be Category D and those for whom Category E will apply, as both will present with the same clinical picture. About the only prognostic indicator is age, as virtually all Category E patients will be relatively young in relation to the degree of destruction present. The important practical distinction between the two categories lies in the fact that Category D patients will respond to therapy, usually within a short period of time.

Thus a Category D patient responds well to plaque control, scaling in selected areas, and sometimes surgery. The Category E patient may practise good plaque control, make visits every 3 months for scaling and root planing in selected areas, may even have surgical removal of pockets and open root planing, yet remains susceptible to the disease process with a constant risk of recurrence.

Indices required

For all patients with sextants scoring 4 or * a complete assessment of probing depths, mobility, bleeding points and overall destruction (including the use of radiographs) is extremely valuable. The response of the indices to therapy from their baseline values will give an indication of which Category the patient belongs to — and thus the prognosis can be estimated with more accuracy.

In order to understand the methods used in data collection and interpretation of the Periodontal Control System the rest of this chapter describes a typical patient undergoing continuing periodontal care. All 4 charts of the system are illustrated with appropriate comments on their use.

Using the Charts

The example which follows is hypothetical, but is based upon experience in general dental surgery. It follows the course of a 32 year old male patient with charts showing the position at first presentation and at 1.2 and 5 years.

Although the example occupies a number of pages with detailed charts the reader is strongly advised to work through these pages with care as they show in-depth the values of the Periodontal Control System in indicating the progress of the disease and the effectiveness of treatment.

A Case History

This hypothetical example charts the progress, on the following pages, of attending for periodontal care.

Fig. 9.1 On initial visit.
Fig. 9.2 1 year later.
Fig. 9.3 2 years following initial visit.
Fig. 9.4 5 years following initial visit.

At each stage a brief description of the clinical situation and a summary treatment plan are presented. Then each of the 4 charts is shown with a synopsis of relevant points which illustrate the application of the charts in the treatment of the patient.

There is no attempt to be comprehensive in this outline, but more to select features of using the charts to help the clinician in his patient care. Also we must stress that the treatment plans suggested are purely for guidance, and a different approach is possible.

Points to OBSERVE or NOTE in the following case study:
The points given below will help identify some of the major advantages to be gained by using these charts.

However, to fully appreciate all of the possible benefits of the Periodontal Control System it is desirable to work through the text in sequence.

Fig. 9.1.a. A quick glance at the D.I., B.I., and CPITN give the clinician an immediate idea of the susceptibility of the patient. Thus the hygienist can have an indication of the patient's clinical condition before seeing him, and can prepare the session accordingly.

Fig. 9.1.c. The shaded representation of the pocket depths shows exactly where the troublesome pockets are and this helps assess the patient's progress in later years (for example Figure 9.4.b on page 111).

Fig. 9.2.a shows how informative the D.I. and B.I. scores are when assessed over a period of time. Compare this with the CPITN scores in the same chart which show a very small improvement. This illustrates the dynamic nature of the D.I. and B.I. which is of much more value in general practice.

Fig. 9.2.d shows how the plaque distribution complements the D.I. where applicable, and the Bleeding Points illustrate the response of the gingivae to flossing in the lower anterior region by the reduction in scores.

Fig. 9.3.b shows how difficult the Index Calculator alone is to show the D.I. and B.I. scores. Compare this with the Monitoring Chart on page 99.

Figure 9.4.a demonstrates the value of recording the areas that have had surgery on the same chart. Note the wealth of factual data gathered on the one sheet showing the long-term record of plaque control scores, gingival health and overall periodontal status. It is possible to gain a general impression of the periodontal response to therapy from this one form over a period of 5 years.

CASE STUDY — Mr J. Jones

First Visit

The CPITN score below indicated that he required special periodontal care and appropriate approval was obtained.

4	4	3
3	2	3

Second Visit

The following indices were taken.

1. Probing depths and bleeding points.
2. Mobility.
3. Periodontal Index.
4. Debris Index and Bleeding Index.

For maximum efficiency the indices were taken in the order stated above. It is important to avoid staining the gingiva with the disclosing tablet until *after* taking the P.I. since the P.I. requires an assessment of frank inflammation.

On completion the 4 forms depicted in Fig. 9.1 were completed.

Most of the problems have occurred in the upper arch. This is an easier arch to treat — especially surgically — so prognosis is improved.

Proposed Treatment Plan

1. Visits with the hygienist now.
2. 3-monthly scaling appointments.
3. Assess for surgery after a year.

Fig. 9.1.a   Monitoring Chart
Points to note on initial examination:

1. *The 6 teeth selected for the D.I. and B.I. include the /5(25) instead of the /4(24) which has been extracted. These teeth have been circled for future reference.*

2. *The CPITN data indicates that the patient falls within Category D. This information also tells the dentist that a probing depth chart will need to be taken, and that the only sextant not requiring individual tooth probing depth charting is the lower anterior sextant.*

3. *The initial D.I. and B.I. scores have been recorded in the "Assessment Section" which can be useful if the patient is to be handed on to the hygienist for all future routine periodontal treatment.*

4. *The patient has a high D.I. (1.3) yet the P.I. is only 3.4. This suggests a good prognosis and the patient can be informed of this on the first visit. If the D.I. had been low (less than 0.6) then the prognosis would have been much worse, and treatment much more difficult. If the P.I. had been above 4.5 in a patient of this age then again the prognosis would have been much worse, (suggesting a Category E).*

Periodontal Control System

NAME __MR J. JONES__ AGE __32__

ASSESSMENT DATE: __23·7·82__

8	7	⑥	5	4	3	2	1	①	2	3	4	⑤	6	7	8
8	7	6	5	④	3	2	①	1	2	3	4	5	⑥	7	8

circle teeth used for DI and BI

CPITN

4	4	3
3	2	3

DEBRIS INDEX __1·3__   BLEEDING INDEX __1·25__

INITIAL TREATMENT

Date	DI	BI
23·7·82	1·3	1·25

Date	DI	BI

Date	PI
23·7·82	3·4

SUGGESTED RECALL INTERVAL

LONG TERM CPITN ASSESSMENT
To be used as desired

Date _____

Date _____

Date _____

Date _____

Date _____

LONG TERM TREATMENT

Date	DI	BI

Date	DI	BI

SURGICAL INTERVENTION

Date _____

Area _____

Date _____

Area _____

Date _____

Area _____

Date _____

Area _____

Date _____

Area _____

Date _____

Area _____

Date _____

Area _____

Date _____

Area _____

79

Fig. 9.1.b   Index Calculator
Points to note on initial examination:

1. *The P.I. section shows how the P.I. has been calculated. The second line and box will be used at the end of the initial treatment (see below for a definition of initial treatment).*

2. *The teeth that had been circled on the Monitoring Chart have been entered and the first D.I. and B.I. calculated.*

3. *This chart is purely to be used as an aid for calculation of P.I., D.I. and B.I. and can be disposed of after it is full.*

For the purposes of these forms initial treatment is regarded as treatment over the first year or two. Usually most patients will either respond to therapy; or else not respond because of a lack of motivation and adequate plaque control. Those that respond may or may not require periodontal surgery.
Thus initial treatment is a period of time of assessment of the patient's motivation, ability to practise adequate plaque control and willingness to partake in a recall programme. By the end of this period the patient may have undergone surgery, but may not. The deciding factor is the opinion of the clinician as to the patient's motivation.

Periodontal Control System

NAME   MR J. JONES

PERIODONTAL INDEX

	6	6	—		6	6	6	6	6	6	—	6			1
8	7	6	5	4	3	2	1	1	2	3	4	5	6	7	8
8	7	6	5	4	3	2	1	1	2	3	4	5	6	7	8
1	6	6	—	0	0	0	0	1	0	0	2	2	6	—	

$$\frac{\text{TOTAL SCORE} \quad 79}{\text{NUMBER OF TEETH} \quad 23} = \boxed{3 \cdot 4}$$

$$\frac{\text{TOTAL SCORE}}{\text{NUMBER OF TEETH}} = \boxed{}$$

DI & BI SCORES

TOOTH	SURFACE	DI	BI	DI	BI	DI	BI	DI	BI	DI	BI	DI	BI	DI	BI
6| (16)	buccal	2	2												
	lingual	1	2												
L| (21)	buccal	2	2												
	lingual	1	0												
|5 (25)	buccal	1	1												
	lingual	1	1												
|6 (36)	buccal	3	2												
	lingual	1	2												
7| (41)	buccal	2	2												
	lingual	0	0												
4| (44)	buccal	2	1												
	lingual	0	0												
TOTAL SCORE		16	15													
INDEX		1·3	1·25													

TOOTH	SURFACE	DI	BI	DI	BI	DI	BI	DI	BI	DI	BI	DI	BI	DI	BI
	buccal														
	lingual														
	buccal														
	lingual														
	buccal														
	lingual														
	buccal														
	lingual														
	buccal														
	lingual														
	buccal														
	lingual														
TOTAL SCORE															
INDEX															

Fig. 9.1.c   Probing Depth Chart
Points to note on initial examination:

1. *Recession has been entered for all teeth to act as a baseline. Probing depths have only been entered in sextants scoring 3 or 4 using the CPITN. This saves on clinical time.*

2. *The shaded areas give an immediate indication of the areas which will require more attention. This saves time when looking at a mass of figures as the chart builds up over time.*

3. *Mobility scores have also been entered for all teeth. This is because some teeth can be mobile in the absence of pockets due to abnormal occlusal stresses.*

Periodontal Control System

NAME **MR J. JONES** AGE **32**

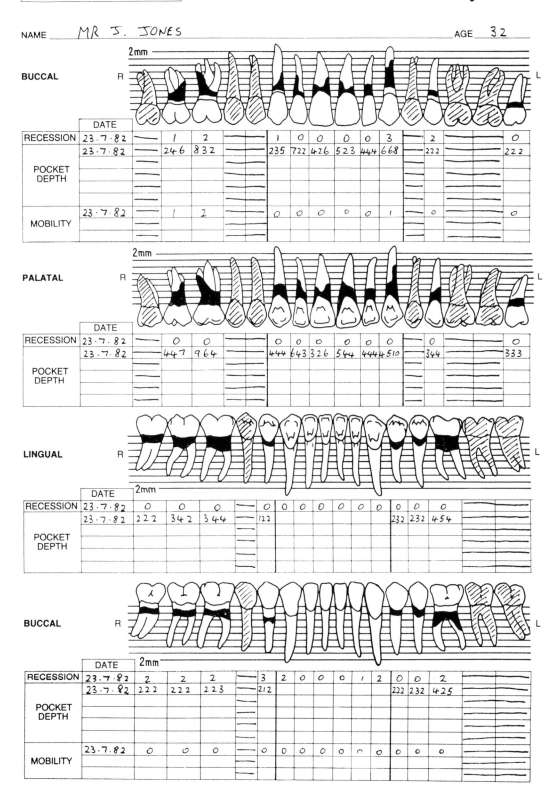

BUCCAL R — L

DATE												
RECESSION 23·7·82		1	2		1	0	0	0	0	3	2	0
23·7·82		246	832		235	722	426	523	444	668	222	222
POCKET DEPTH												
MOBILITY 23·7·82		1	2		0	0	0	0	0	1	0	0

PALATAL R — L

DATE												
RECESSION 23·7·82		0	0		0	0	0	0	0	0	0	0
23·7·82		447	964		444	643	326	544	444	510	344	333
POCKET DEPTH												

LINGUAL R — L

DATE												
RECESSION 23·7·82	0	0	0		0	0	0	0	0	0	0	0	0
23·7·82	222	342	344		122						232	232	454
POCKET DEPTH												

BUCCAL R — L

DATE												
RECESSION 23·7·82	2	2	2		3	2	0	0	0	1	2	0	0	2
23·7·82	222	222	223		212						222	232	425
POCKET DEPTH												
MOBILITY 23·7·82	0	0	0		0	0	0	0	0	⌐	0	0	0

Fig. 9.1.d   Distribution Chart
Points to note on initial examination:

1. *The plaque distribution chart has not been used at all for this patient. This chart is more often used as an aid to motivation and so is more likely to be effective later in the treatment.*

2. *The bleeding distribution chart shows generalised bleeding throughout the mouth.*

84

Periodontal Control System

NAME ___MR J, JONES___ AGE __32__

PLAQUE DISTRIBUTION

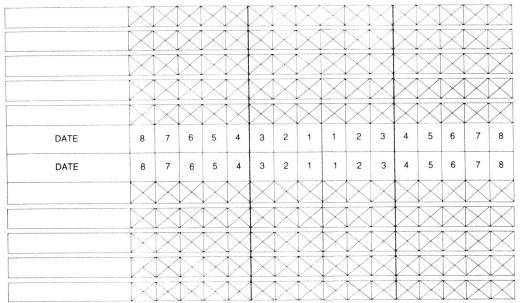

DATE	8	7	6	5	4	3	2	1	1	2	3	4	5	6	7	8
DATE	8	7	6	5	4	3	2	1	1	2	3	4	5	6	7	8

BLEEDING POINTS DISTRIBUTION

23.7.82																
DATE	8	7	6	5	4	3	2	1	1	2	3	4	5	6	7	8
DATE	8	7	6	5	4	3	2	1	1	2	3	4	5	6	7	8
23.7.82																

After 1 Year

Fig. 9.2 shows the charts after one year, indicating the progress that has been made since the first visit. Comparison of these charts with the charts in Fig. 9.1 will give an idea of how easy it is to measure progress and the patient's reaction to therapy.

The Monitoring Chart shows a rather slow compliance with plaque control instruction and erratic behaviour of the scores. The Bleeding Index has tended to follow the plaque scores, suggesting that once the plaque is brought under continuous control the inflammation will respond.

Clearly in this patient the response to plaque control is all important. At this point the plaque distribution chart might be completed, on the basis that the extra motivational effect may justify the time involved.

Note how easy it is to interpret the D.I. and B.I. scores when they are set out in tabular form (as in the Monitoring Chart). A glance at the Index Calculator sheet where the scores are set out in a straight line illustrates the point. Again it is worth noting that the Index Calculator Sheet is intended only to help calculate D.I., B.I.

and P.I. scores, not to provide a permanent record.

On completion the 4 forms are shown in Fig. 9.2.

The dates on the Monitoring Chart give an indication that the patient has attended for 2 appointments with the hygienist for scaling and plaque control instruction within a three-week period, followed by an interval of three months before a third appointment. This is evidence that whilst he may not yet be motivated towards good plaque control, he is motivated enough to attend for the treatment.

Despite this he has not yet succeeded in maintaining a good plaque level consistently. So, although deep pockets persist, surgery cannot be considered yet.

There is a general trend of reduction in the probing depths. This is data which can be used to encourage the patient.

Proposed Treatment Plan Now

1. Continue with the hygienist appointments.
2. Maintain a maximum recall interval of three months.
3. Assess for surgery as soon as the plaque levels stabilise.

Fig. 9.2.a   Monitoring Chart
Points to note after 1 year:

1. *The dates on the Monitoring Chart give an indication that the patient has attended for 2 appointments with the hygienist for scaling and plaque control instruction within a three-week period, followed by an interval of three months before a third appointment. This is evidence that whilst he may not yet be motivated towards good plaque control, he is motivated enough to attend for treatment.*

2. *In August 1983 after a period of about 4 months only there was a worsening of the D.I. score from 0.5 to 1.1. This was followed by a score of 1.0 in December after another 4 months. Thus the hygienist thought a reassessment advisable and the patient attended after a month when the CPITN, probing depths and bleeding distribution were all recorded again.*

3. *The CPITN score showed an improvement in 2 sextants, upper left posterior sextant and lower right posterior sextant.*

4. *Because of the deterioration in plaque control the dentist thought this patient had not yet stabilised (from a plaque control viewpoint) and thus estimated the patient was not yet ready for any surgery. This means initial treatment is still continuing.*

Periodontal Control System

NAME _MR J. JONES_ AGE _32 34_

ASSESSMENT DATE: | 23 · 7 · 82 |

| 8 | 7 | ⑥ | 5 | 4 | 3 | 2 | 1 | ① | 2 | 3 | 4 | ⑤ | 6 | 7 | 8 |
| 8 | 7 | 6 | 5 | ④ | 3 | 2 | ① | 1 | 2 | 3 | 4 | 5 | ⑥ | 7 | 8 |

circle teeth used for DI and BI

CPITN

| 4 | 4 | 3 |
| 3 | 2 | 3 |

DEBRIS INDEX | 1·3 | BLEEDING INDEX | 1·25 |

INITIAL TREATMENT

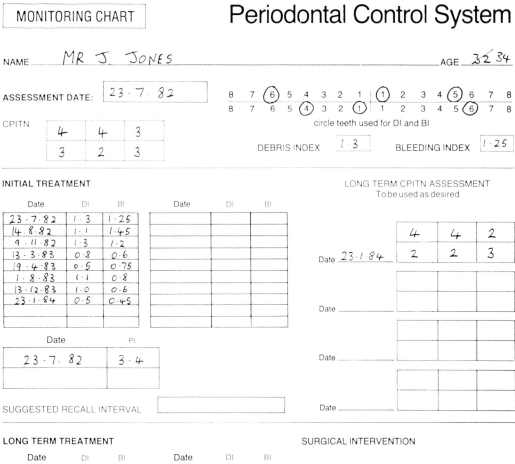

Date	DI	BI	Date	DI	BI
23·7·82	1·3	1·25			
14·8·82	1·1	1·45			
9·11·82	1·3	1·2			
13·3·83	0·8	0·6			
19·4·83	0·5	0·75			
1·8·83	1·1	0·8			
13·12·83	1·0	0·6			
23·1·84	0·5	0·45			

Date		PI
23·7·82		3·4

SUGGESTED RECALL INTERVAL [   ]

LONG TERM CPITN ASSESSMENT
To be used as desired

| 4 | 4 | 2 |
| 2 | 2 | 3 |

Date _23·1·84_

Date _____

Date _____

Date _____

Date _____

LONG TERM TREATMENT

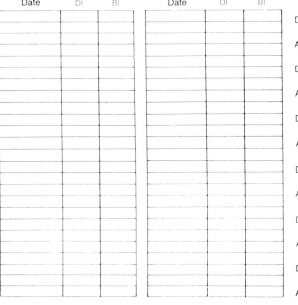

Date	DI	BI	Date	DI	BI

SURGICAL INTERVENTION

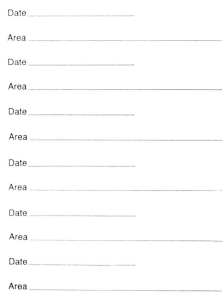

Date _____

Area _____

Date _____

Area _____

Date _____

Area _____

Date _____

Area _____

Date _____

Area _____

Date _____

Area _____

89

Fig. 9.2.b Index Calculator
Points to note after 1 year:

1. *The number of figures on this chart are beginning to make the D.I. and B.I. scores difficult to interpret. This is why this form is not used to replace the Monitoring Chart.*

INDEX CALCULATOR

Periodontal Control System

NAME MR J. JONES

PERIODONTAL INDEX

—	6	6	—	—	6	6	6	6	6	6	—	6	—	—	1
8	7	6	5	4	3	2	1	1	2	3	4	5	6	7	8
8	7	6	5	4	3	2	1	1	2	3	4	5	6	7	8
1	6	6	—	0	0	0	0	1	0	0	2	2	6	—	—

TOTAL SCORE 79 / NUMBER OF TEETH 23 = 3.4

TOTAL SCORE / NUMBER OF TEETH =

DI & BI SCORES

TOOTH	SURFACE	SCORE DI	BI	DI	BI	DI	BI	DI	BI	DI	BI	DI	BI	DI	BI
6| (16)	buccal	2	2	2	2	2	2	1	0	0	0	1	1	1	1
	lingual	1	2	1	1	1	2	2	1	1	1	2	2	2	1
|1 (21)	buccal	2	2	1	2	1	1	1	1	0	1	1	1	1	1
	lingual	1	0	1	2	1	1	1	1	0	1	1	1	1	1
|5 (25)	buccal	1	1	1	1	1	1	1	0	0	0	1	0	1	0
	lingual	1	1	1	1	2	1	1	1	1	2	1	1	1	1
|6 (36)	buccal	3	2	2	2	1	1	1	0	1	1	1	1	0	1
	lingual	1	2	1	2	2	2	1	1	2	1	3	1	2	1
1| (41)	buccal	2	2	1	1	1	1	0	1	1	0	1	1	1	0
	lingual	0	0	0	1	1	1	0	1	0	1	0	0	1	0
4| (44)	buccal	2	1	2	2	1	1	1	1	1	1	1	1	1	1
	lingual	0	0	0	0	1	0	0	0	0	0	0	0	0	0
TOTAL SCORE		16	15	13	17	15	14	10	8	7	9	13	10	12	8
INDEX		1·3	1·25	1·1	1·45	1·3	1·2	0·8	0·6	0·5	0·75	1·1	0·8	1·0	0·6

TOOTH	SURFACE	SCORE DI	BI	DI	BI	DI	BI	DI	BI	DI	BI	DI	BI	DI	BI
6| (16)	buccal	1	1												
	lingual	1	1												
|1 (21)	buccal	0	1												
	lingual	1	0												
|5 (25)	buccal	0	0												
	lingual	1	1												
|6 (36)	buccal	0	0												
	lingual	2	1												
1| (41)	buccal	0	0												
	lingual	0	0												
4| (44)	buccal	0	0												
	lingual	0	0												
TOTAL SCORE		6	5												
INDEX		0·5	0·45												

Fig. 9.2.c Probing Depth Chart
Points to note after 1 year:

1. *There is a general trend of reduction in the probing depths. This is data which can be used to encourage the patient.*

2. *The shaded areas on the Probing Depth Chart make it much easier to identify the danger areas immediately.*

3. *Much less of the chart needs scoring on an individual tooth basis because the CPITN score has identified the areas where some pocketing is present. This is a great saving in clinical time.*

Periodontal Control System

NAME MR J. JONES   AGE 3/2 34

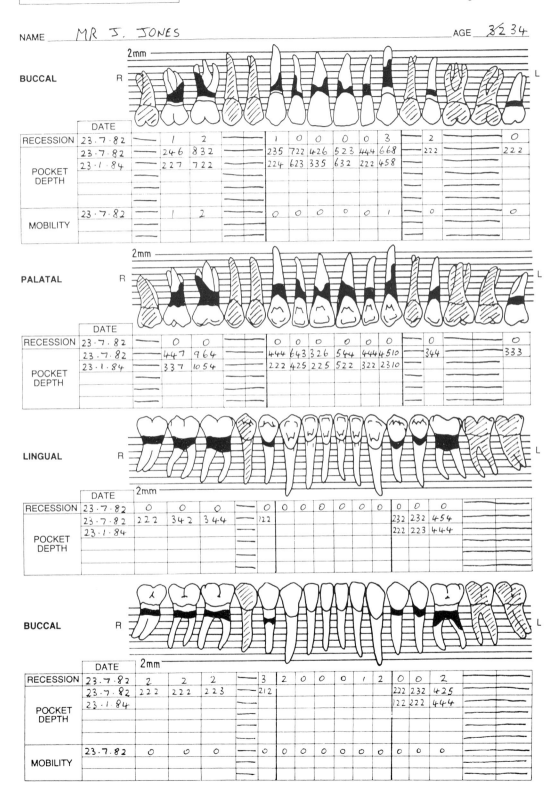

BUCCAL R   L

	DATE														
RECESSION	23·7·82		1	2		1	0	0	0	0	3		2		0
POCKET DEPTH	23·7·82		246	832		235	722	426	523	444	668		222		222
	23·1·84		227	722		224	623	335	632	222	458				
MOBILITY	23·7·82		1	2		0	0	0	0	0	1		0		0

PALATAL R   L

	DATE														
RECESSION	23·7·82		0	0		0	0	0	0	0	0		0		0
POCKET DEPTH	23·7·82		447	964		444	643	326	544	444	510		344		333
	23·1·84		337	1054		222	425	225	522	322	2310				

LINGUAL R   L

	DATE														
RECESSION	23·7·82	0	0	0		0	0	0	0	0	0	0	0	0	0
POCKET DEPTH	23·7·82	222	342	344		122						232	232	454	
	23·1·84											222	223	444	

BUCCAL R   L

	DATE														
RECESSION	23·7·82	2	2	2		3	2	0	0	0	1	2	0	0	2
POCKET DEPTH	23·7·82	222	222	223		212							222	232	425
	23·1·84												122	222	444
MOBILITY	23·7·82	0	0	0		0	0	0	0	0	0	0	0	0	

Fig. 9.2.d   Distribution Chart
Points to note after 1 year:

1. *Normally the Bleeding Points Chart is only completed at the same time as the probing depths. However, in this case the hygienist took an additional charting (on 9.11.82) to try to help motivate the patient by showing him the improvement.*

2. *When the patient showed a worsening of the D.I. the hygienist used the plaque distribution chart to identify the areas causing concern. This was taken again after an improvement to act as a reinforcement for motivation.*

Periodontal Control System

NAME __MR J. JONES__   AGE __3̶2̶ 34__

PLAQUE DISTRIBUTION

	8	7	6	5	4	3	2	1	1	2	3	4	5	6	7	8
23 · 1 · 84																
13 · 12 · 83																
DATE	8	7	6	5	4	3	2	1	1	2	3	4	5	6	7	8
DATE	8	7	6	5	4	3	2	1	1	2	3	4	5	6	7	8
13 · 12 · 83																
23 · 1 · 84																

BLEEDING POINTS DISTRIBUTION

	8	7	6	5	4	3	2	1	1	2	3	4	5	6	7	8
23 · 1 · 84																
9 · 11 · 82																
23 · 7 · 82																
DATE	8	7	6	5	4	3	2	1	1	2	3	4	5	6	7	8
DATE	8	7	6	5	4	3	2	1	1	2	3	4	5	6	7	8
23 · 7 · 82																
9 · 11 · 82																
23 · 1 · 84																

95

After 2 Years

Fig. 9.3 contains all the information obtained in the two years following the first visit. The patient has responded to plaque control (as the D.I. scores demonstrate vividly) so that he can be considered to have reached a stage of stabilisation.

Thus the date of 'primary stabilisation' is recorded on the Monitoring Chart, together with an indication of the time spent achieving this. Also the new P.I. is recorded (showing excellent improvement) and a recommended recall interval chosen and recorded.

In this case the recall interval has been set at 4 months. This was chosen partly in response to the patient's wishes (a change of job means he finds it more difficult to attend) and partly because the dentist felt this to be the best interval (ideally to be kept at 3 months).

The four forms on completion of the two years are illustrated in Fig. 9.3.

The Probing Depths Chart illustrates that there are still some deep pockets which are not responding to conventional therapy. These tissues are still bleeding (see the Bleeding Points Chart) giving us a positive indication for periodontal surgery.

The excellent D.I. scores over the period of 1 year also show that the patient is now motivated. Combining these figures with the presence of the deep bleeding pockets gives all the information needed to make a decision regarding surgery. It is not a difficult decision — for the monitoring charts make it obvious there is little choice once the patient agrees. This subject is covered more fully in Chapter 11.

Proposed Treatment Plan Now

1. Carry out a surgical procedure (Inverse bevel flap and open root planing) in 1 area (say the 43 to 33 area) and monitor the result prior to deciding whether to use surgery in the upper right sextant.

2. Continue with the hygienist appointments.

Fig. 9.3.a   Monitoring Chart
Points to note after 2 years:

1. *The fact that the patient has now maintained a score below 0.5 for D.I. for 12 months and attended at 3-monthly intervals shows a high degree of motivation. Thus this patient can be said to have reached the end of initial treatment.*
Notice how easy it is to monitor the plaque levels against the bleeding levels over a period of time.

2. *The CPITN score shows further improvement.*

3. *The P.I. is also taken again, showing an overall improvement.*

4. *The box suggesting a recall interval acts as a general reminder to both dentist and patient in the future.*

98

Periodontal Control System

NAME _MR J. JONES_   AGE _32 34_

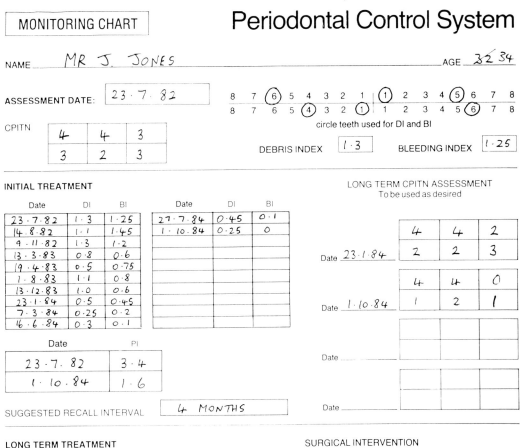

ASSESSMENT DATE: | 23 · 7 · 82 |

| 8 | 7 | (6) | 5 | 4 | 3 | 2 | 1 | (1) | 2 | 3 | 4 | (5) | 6 | 7 | 8 |
| 8 | 7 | 6 | 5 | (4) | 3 | 2 | (1) | 1 | 2 | 3 | 4 | 5 | (6) | 7 | 8 |

circle teeth used for DI and BI

CPITN

| 4 | 4 | 3 |
| 3 | 2 | 3 |

DEBRIS INDEX | 1·3 | BLEEDING INDEX | 1·25 |

INITIAL TREATMENT

Date	DI	BI
23·7·82	1·3	1·25
14·8·82	1·1	1·45
9·11·82	1·3	1·2
13·3·83	0·8	0·6
19·4·83	0·5	0·75
1·8·83	1·1	0·8
13·12·83	1·0	0·6
23·1·84	0·5	0·45
7·3·84	0·25	0·2
16·6·84	0·3	0·1

Date	DI	BI
27·7·84	0·45	0·1
1·10·84	0·25	0

Date	PI
23·7·82	3·4
1·10·84	1·6

SUGGESTED RECALL INTERVAL | 4 MONTHS |

LONG TERM CPITN ASSESSMENT
To be used as desired

| 4 | 4 | 2 |
| 2 | 2 | 3 |

Date _23·1·84_

| 4 | 4 | 0 |
| 1 | 2 | 1 |

Date _1·10·84_

Date _____

Date _____

Date _____

LONG TERM TREATMENT

Date	DI	BI	Date	DI	BI

SURGICAL INTERVENTION

Date _____

Area _____

Date _____

Area _____

Date _____

Area _____

Date _____

Area _____

Date _____

Area _____

Date _____

Area _____

Figure 9.3.b   Index Calculator

1. It should be noted that this chart is nearing the end of its life. Note how the P.I. and the B.I. and D.I. scores have been calculated.

Periodontal Control System

NAME __MR J. JONES__

PERIODONTAL INDEX

—	6	6	—	—	O	6	6	6	O	6	—	—	O	—	1
—	6	6	—	—	6	6	6	6	6	6	—	—	6	—	1
8	7	6	5	4	3	2	1	1	2	3	4	5	6	7	8
8	7	6	5	4	3	2	1	1	2	3	4	5	6	7	8
1	6	6	—	O	O	O	O	1	O	O	2	2	6	—	—
1	O	O	—	O	O	O	O	O	O	O	O	O	O	—	—

TOTAL SCORE __79__ / NUMBER OF TEETH 23 = [3.4]

TOTAL SCORE __38__ / NUMBER OF TEETH 23 = [1.6]

DI & BI SCORES

TOOTH	SURFACE	DI	BI	DI	BI	DI	BI	DI	BI	DI	BI	DI	BI	DI	BI
6| (16)	buccal	2	2	2	2	2	2	1	0	0	0	1	1	1	1
	lingual	1	2	1	1	1	2	2	1	1	1	2	2	2	1
L| (21)	buccal	2	2	1	2	1	1	1	1	0	1	1	1	1	1
	lingual	1	0	1	2	1	1	1	1	0	1	1	1	1	1
|5 (25)	buccal	1	1	1	1	1	1	1	0	0	0	1	0	1	0
	lingual	1	1	1	1	2	1	1	1	1	2	1	1	1	1
|6 (36)	buccal	3	2	2	2	1	1	1	0	1	1	1	1	0	1
	lingual	1	2	1	2	2	2	1	1	2	1	3	1	2	1
|7 (41)	buccal	2	2	1	1	1	1	0	1	1	0	1	1	1	0
	lingual	0	0	0	1	1	1	0	1	0	1	0	0	1	0
4| (44)	buccal	2	1	2	2	1	1	1	1	1	1	1	1	1	1
	lingual	0	0	0	0	1	0	0	0	0	0	0	0	0	0
TOTAL SCORE		16	15	13	17	15	14	10	8	7	9	13	10	12	8
INDEX		1.3	1.25	1.1	1.45	1.3	1.2	0.8	0.6	0.5	0.75	1.1	0.8	1.0	0.6

TOOTH	SURFACE	DI	BI	DI	BI	DI	BI	DI	BI	DI	BI	DI	BI	DI	BI
6| (16)	buccal	1	1	0	0	0	0	0	0	0	0				
	lingual	1	1	1	0	1	0	1	0	1	0				
L| (21)	buccal	0	1	0	0	0	0	0	0	0	0				
	lingual	1	0	0	0	0	1	0	0	0	0				
|5 (25)	buccal	0	0	0	0	0	0	0	0	0	0				
	lingual	1	1	1	1	1	0	2	0	0	0				
|6 (36)	buccal	0	0	0	0	0	0	0	0	0	0				
	lingual	2	1	1	0	1	0	0	0	0	0				
|7 (41)	buccal	0	0	0	0	0	0	0	0	0	0				
	lingual	0	0	0	1	0	0	1	1	1	0				
4| (44)	buccal	0	0	0	0	0	0	0	0	0	0				
	lingual	0	0	0	0	1	0	1	0	1	0				
TOTAL SCORE		6	5	3	2	4	1	5	1	3	0				
INDEX		0.5	0.45	0.25	0.2	0.3	0.1	0.45	0.1	0.25	0				

Fig. 9.3.c Probing Depth Chart
Points to note after 2 years:

1. *The CPITN score shows that now the only areas that need measuring are the upper anterior and right sextants. Pockets in these areas show a general improvement except for the deeper pockets – some of which are deepening.*

2. *The Probing Depths Chart illustrates that there are still some deep pockets which are not responding to conventional therapy. These tissues are still bleeding (see the Bleeding Points Chart) giving us a positive indication for periodontal surgery.*

3. *The excellent D.I. scores over the period of 1 year also show that the patient is now motivated. Combining these figures with the presence of the deep bleeding pockets gives all the information needed to make a decision regarding surgery. It is not a difficult decision – for the monitoring charts make it obvious there is little choice once the patient agrees.*

4. *Mobility scores also show an improvement. This patient is well stabilised and the periodontal disease is responding to plaque control.*

Periodontal Control System

PROBING DEPTH CHART

NAME MR J. JONES   AGE 3̶2̶ 34

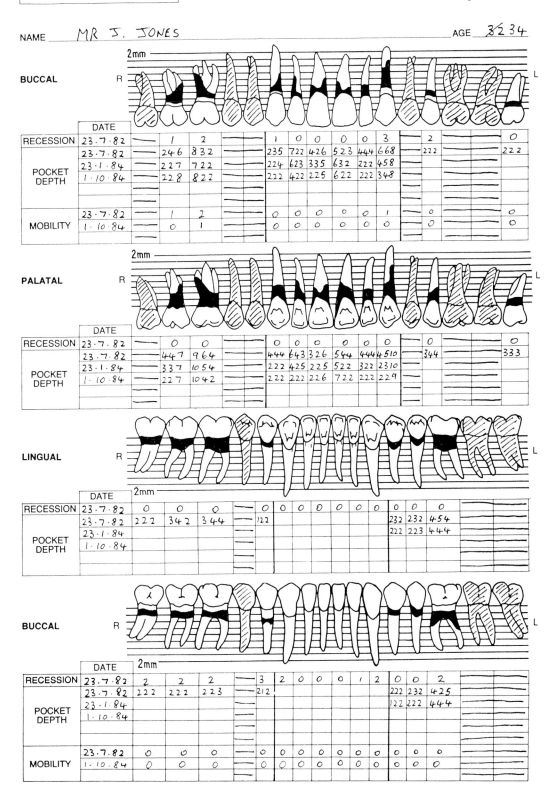

BUCCAL — R ... L — 2mm

	DATE															
RECESSION	23·7·82		1	2		1	0	0	0	0	3		2			0
POCKET DEPTH	23·7·82		246	832		235	722	426	523	444	668		222			222
	23·1·84		227	722		224	623	335	632	222	458					
	1·10·84		228	822		222	422	225	622	222	348					
MOBILITY	23·7·82		1	2		0	0	0	0	0	1		0			0
	1·10·84		0	1		0	0	0	0	0	0		0			0

PALATAL — R ... L — 2mm

	DATE															
RECESSION	23·7·82		0	0		0	0	0	0	0	0		0			0
POCKET DEPTH	23·7·82		447	964		444	643	326	544	444	510		344			333
	23·1·84		337	1054		222	425	225	522	322	2310					
	1·10·84		227	1042		222	222	226	722	222	229					

LINGUAL — R ... L — 2mm

	DATE															
RECESSION	23·7·82	0	0	0		0	0	0	0	0	0	0	0	0	0	
POCKET DEPTH	23·7·82	222	342	344		122							232	232	454	
	23·1·84													222	223	444
	1·10·84															

BUCCAL — R ... L — 2mm

	DATE															
RECESSION	23·7·82	2	2	2		3	2	0	0	1	2	0	0	2		
POCKET DEPTH	23·7·82	222	222	223		212							222	232	425	
	23·1·84													122	222	444
	1·10·84															
MOBILITY	23·7·82	0	0	0		0	0	0	0	0	0	0	0	0	0	
	1·10·84	0	0	0		0	0	0	0	0	0	0	0	0	0	

Fig. 9.3.d   Distribution Chart

1. It should be noted that the bleeding points are linked to areas with deep pockets (as would be expected). Compare the bleeding points with the Probing Depth Chart.

Periodontal Control System

NAME __MR J. JONES__   AGE __32 34__

PLAQUE DISTRIBUTION

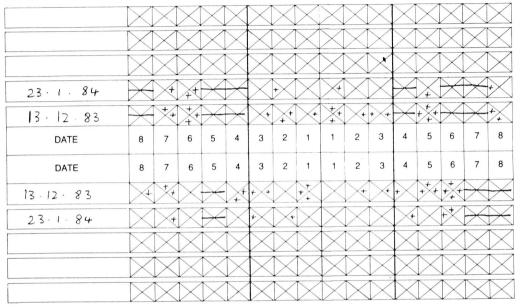

23 · 1 · 84																
13 · 12 · 83																
DATE	8	7	6	5	4	3	2	1	1	2	3	4	5	6	7	8
DATE	8	7	6	5	4	3	2	1	1	2	3	4	5	6	7	8
13 · 12 · 83																
23 · 1 · 84																

BLEEDING POINTS DISTRIBUTION

1 · 10 · 84																
23 · 1 · 84																
9 · 11 · 82																
23 · 7 · 82																
DATE	8	7	6	5	4	3	2	1	1	2	3	4	5	6	7	8
DATE	8	7	6	5	4	3	2	1	1	2	3	4	5	6	7	8
23 · 7 · 82																
9 · 11 · 82																
23 · 1 · 84																
1 · 10 · 84																

105

After 5 Years

Now that the disease has been arrested and treated by surgery we can look ahead to see how the charts monitor over the longterm. The only charts shown in Fig. 9.4 are the Probing Depth Chart and the Monitoring Chart (although the others are still being kept).

Surgery has been carried out and there has been a dramatic reduction in pocket depth (but note also the increased recession following the surgery).

The 2 relevant forms are shown in Fig. 9.4.

The Monitoring Chart still gives an excellent longterm picture of the disease process over many years. As all the information is on the one page, this style of information is of much greater value to the dentist and hygienist *in this form* than in a number of smaller charts which need to be continually checked.

Having the surgical areas indicated together with the dates when the procedures were carried out is also invaluable when talking to the patient. There is an immediate guide as to where and when surgery was performed. There is no need to search back through several years of notes.

The patient did in fact have 6-monthly recalls with the hygienist for a spell (between April 1986 — June 1987) but as soon as the increased B.I. was spotted this interval was shortened again.

Proposed Treatment Plan Now

1. Continue with the hygienist appointments.

Fig. 9.4.a   Monitoring Chart
Points to note after 5 years:

1. *The Monitoring Chart still gives an excellent longterm picture of the disease process over many years. As all the information is on the one page, this style of information is of much greater value to the dentist and hygienist* in this form *than in a number of smaller charts which need to be continually checked.*

2. *Note the sudden increase in B.I. scores in June 1987, with a slight decrease in D.I. scores. The patient could be going through a 'burst' of disease activity. This situation prompted the CPITN which highlighted 2 areas of deeper pocketing and potential danger. Note that the lower left sextant had originally improved but was now deteriorating again.*

2. *Having the surgical areas indicated together with the dates when the procedures were carried out is also invaluable when talking to the patient. There is an immediate guide as to where and when surgery was performed. There is no need to search back through several years of notes.*

3. *The patient did in fact have 6-monthly recalls with the hygienist for a spell (between April 1986 – June 1987) but as soon as the increased B.I. was spotted this interval was shortened again.*

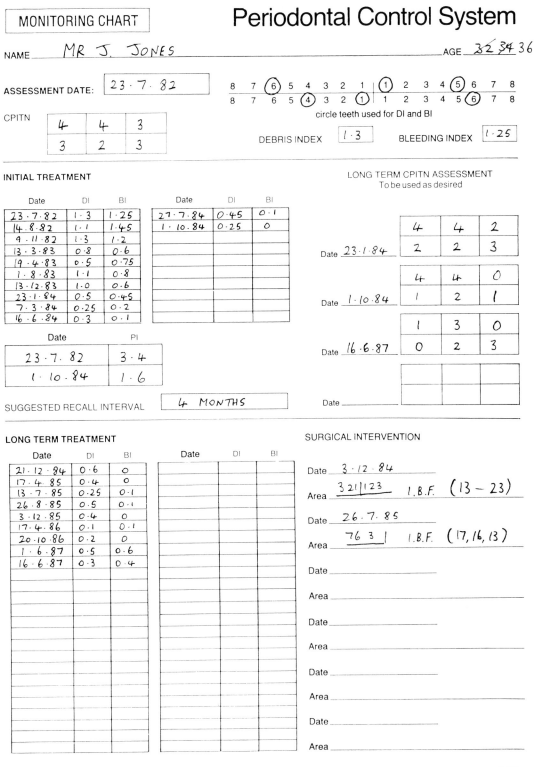

Periodontal Control System

MONITORING CHART

NAME MR J. JONES   AGE 32 34 36

ASSESSMENT DATE: 23·7·82

| | 8 | 7 | ⑥ | 5 | 4 | 3 | 2 | 1 | ① | 2 | 3 | 4 | ⑤ | 6 | 7 | 8 |
| | 8 | 7 | 6 | 5 | ④ | 3 | 2 | ① | 1 | 2 | 3 | 4 | 5 | ⑥ | 7 | 8 |

circle teeth used for DI and BI

CPITN

4	4	3
3	2	3

DEBRIS INDEX 1·3   BLEEDING INDEX 1·25

INITIAL TREATMENT

Date	DI	BI	Date	DI	BI
23·7·82	1·3	1·25	27·7·84	0·45	0·1
14·8·82	1·1	1·45	1·10.84	0·25	0
9·11·82	1·3	1·2			
13·3·83	0·8	0·6			
19·4·83	0·5	0·75			
1·8·83	1·1	0·8			
13·12·83	1·0	0·6			
23·1·84	0·5	0·45			
7·3·84	0·25	0·2			
16·6·84	0·3	0·1			

Date	PI
23·7·82	3·4
1·10·84	1·6

SUGGESTED RECALL INTERVAL   4 MONTHS

LONG TERM CPITN ASSESSMENT
To be used as desired

Date 23·1·84

4	4	2
2	2	3

Date 1·10·84

4	4	0
1	2	1

Date 16·6·87

1	3	0
0	2	3

Date _____

LONG TERM TREATMENT

Date	DI	BI	Date	DI	BI
21·12·84	0·6	0			
17·4·85	0·4	0			
13·7·85	0·25	0·1			
26·8·85	0·5	0·1			
3·12·85	0·4	0			
17·4·86	0·1	0·1			
20·10·86	0·2	0			
1·6·87	0·5	0·6			
16·6·87	0·3	0·4			

SURGICAL INTERVENTION

Date 3·12·84

Area 3 2 1 | 1 2 3   I.B.F. (13 – 23)

Date 26·7·85

Area 7 6 3 | 1   I.B.F. (17, 16, 13)

Date _____

Area _____

Date _____

Area _____

Date _____

Area _____

Date _____

Area _____

109

Fig. 9.4.b   Probing Depth Chart
Points to note after 5 years:

1. *Surgery has been carried out and there has been a dramatic reduction in pocket depth (but note also the increased recession following the surgery).*

2. *The Probing Depths Chart contains so much information it could be confusing and it might have been better to start a new chart following the surgery. However it is still possible to see the relevant spots and also to check the danger areas.*

3. *Just completing sextants scoring 3 and 4 in the CPITN has made it easier to isolate areas which require attention.*

Periodontal Control System

NAME MR J. JONES AGE 32 34 36

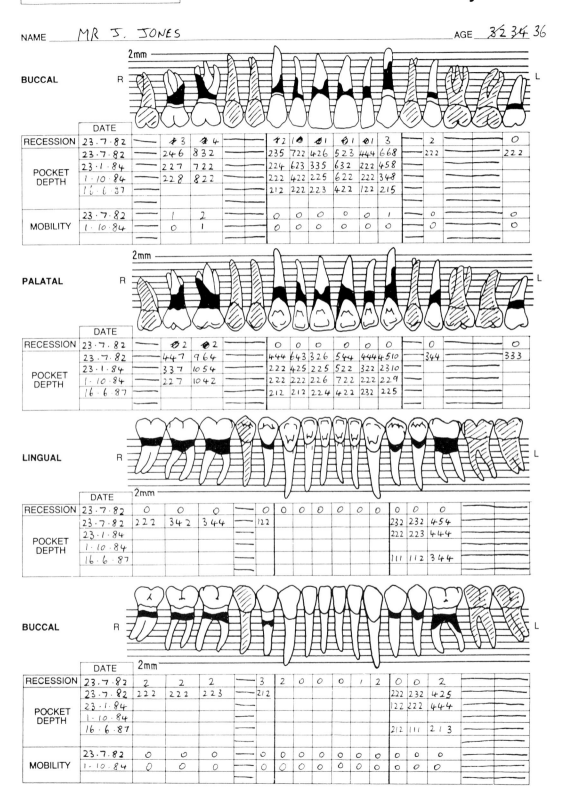

BUCCAL R — L (2mm)

	DATE													
RECESSION	23·7·82	—	↓3	↓4	—	↓2 1↓	↓1	↓1	↓1	3	—	2	—	0
POCKET DEPTH	23·7·82	—	246	832	—	235 722 426	523 444 668	—	222	—	222
	23·1·84	—	227	722	—	224 623 335	632 222 458				
	1·10·84	—	228	822	—	222 422 225	622 222 348				
	16·6·87	—			—	212 222 223	422 122 215				
MOBILITY	23·7·82	—	1	2	—	0 0 0	0 0 1	—	0	—	0
	1·10·84	—	0	1	—	0 0 0	0 0 0	—	0	—	0

PALATAL R — L (2mm)

	DATE									
RECESSION	23·7·82	—	↓2	↓2	—	0 0 0	0 0 0	—	0	—	0
POCKET DEPTH	23·7·82	—	447	964	—	444 643 326	544 444 510	—	344	—	333
	23·1·84	—	337	1054	—	222 425 225	522 322 2310			
	1·10·84	—	227	1042	—	222 222 226	722 222 229			
	16·6·87	—			—	212 212 224	422 232 225			

LINGUAL R — L (2mm)

	DATE											
RECESSION	23·7·82	0	0	0	—	0 0 0 0 0 0 0	0 0 0		
POCKET DEPTH	23·7·82	222	342	344	—	122		232 232 454
	23·1·84				—			222 223 444
	1·10·84				—			
	16·6·87				—			111 112 344

BUCCAL R — L (2mm)

	DATE													
RECESSION	23·7·82	2	2	2	—	3	2	0	0	0	1	2	0	0	2
POCKET DEPTH	23·7·82	222	222	223	—	212						222 232 425
	23·1·84				—							122 222 444
	1·10·84				—							
	16·6·87				—							212 111 213
MOBILITY	23·7·82	0	0	0	—	0 0 0 0 0 0	0 0 0		
	1·10·84	0	0	0	—	0 0 0 0 0 0	0 0 0		

Summary

The preceding pages have shown how the monitoring forms can be used to follow a patient from his initial visit through several years of continuous therapy.

It is easy to see how much information can be obtained by studying the forms. This is a great saver of clinical time and means that decisions regarding the next stage in treatment based on a wealth of information can be made.

But the bonus from all this information is that the dentist can read through the forms prior to seeing the patient or during discussion with the hygienist, and with little effort, know all he needs to know about that patient to make an informed decision regarding future treatment.

Chapter 10

Coping with Category E Patients

Some patients are more susceptible to periodontal disease and the disease process continues despite attempts to control plaque by both the patient and dentist. It may not be possible to distinguish these patients from Category D patients for several months after the initial examination, although a provisional diagnosis can be made in cases where there seems to be excessive bone loss and inflammation in the presence of relatively low levels of plaque, especially in younger patients.

These patients can be classified as Category E and require special attention once they are identified. This chapter discusses some of the ways in which the general practitioner can help them.

Cases of Juvenile Periodontitis

Juvenile periodontitis is now recognised as a specific disease separate from generalised periodontitis. Previously termed periodontosis (due to the belief it was a degenerative disorder because of the observation of low levels of inflammation) juvenile periodontitis tends to affect older children and young adults. The traditional clinical picture is one of infrabony pocketing around the incisors and first molars with a lack of gingival inflammation, followed by a rapidly progressing loss of bone leading to loss of the affected teeth. Eventually the process spreads to the remainder of the dentition. It is now believed that the disease is initiated by the combination of invasion by particular strains of bacteria (*Actinobacillus actinomycetemcomitans* and *Capnocytophaga*) and a defect in the immune response. Whether the bacteria cause the defect in the immunological response or the immunological defect allows the bacteria to invade is not known, but it is now clear that juvenile periodontitis is a different disease from adult generalised periodontitis.

Treatment revolves around intensive plaque control, scaling and root planing, surgery where applicable, and a maintenance programme with frequent visits to control the disease. In some cases courses of tetracycline lasting 3 weeks have contributed to its control. When a general practitioner encounters such cases referral to a specialist centre is advised, but if that is impossible then a pattern of care along the principles outlined in this book may control the disease. In fact these patients often respond to the same programme of care as Category E patients described later in this chapter.

113

Antibiotics and Antiseptics

If a patient is not responding to plaque control and scaling of selected areas the possibility of using an antibacterial agent appears attractive. The ability to satisfy the patient's demands for treatment can overcome the practitioner's natural caution however, and a balanced outlook is essential.

The use of tetracycline in juvenile periodontitis has already been mentioned (1) and can also be used to control the Category E type of disease. Metronidazole is a particularly effective antimicrobial agent in the control of acute ulcerative gingivitis, but not unfortunately in juvenile periodontitis. A recent study (2) has shown that metronidazole is more effective in patients with severe disease suggesting a link between the causative agent and the type of periodontitis. Topical application of antibiotics penicillin and erythromycin can be effective but this method suffers from difficulties in resistance and sensitivity, and most studies show that the effect is only temporary.

The other effective chemical agent is chlorhexidene gluconate which has been found to reduce supragingival plaque levels when administered as a mouthwash twice a day in a concentration of 0.2 per cent. There are certain side-effects to the use of this agent, notably staining of the teeth and in some cases strange taste sensations. Rinsing with chlorhexidene is effective due to the fact that it is a cation and as such binds quickly to proteinaceous tooth deposits and salivary protein, from which it is slowly released to give a prolonged effect. Other antibacterial mouthwashes tend to retain their effectiveness for extremely short periods and thus are relatively ineffective although recent work has found Listerine (eucalyptol), thymol, methyl salicylate and menthol) to retard the development of supragingival plaque.[3] [4]

It is probably most unwise to rely upon chlorhexidene for long term plaque control, but short courses of treatment (a few weeks at most) are helpful in the Category E patient. Because the effect is supragingival only, attempts have been made to teach patients a form of subgingival irrigation but this has had limited success. This is almost certainly due to the inherent difficulty in inserting a blunt syringe needle into pockets within one's mouth, and the motivation required by the patient is considerable.

When using oral irrigators with chlorhexidene the concentration must be reduced (0.02% is recommended). The effect appears to remain supragingival only. At present the oral irrigator can be considered as a useful tool for some patients in conveying the antibacterial agent to the periodontal tissues, and further work may show this to be an effective adjunct in the control of Category E patients.

The Category E Regimen

As already mentioned Category E patients can be identified only by the response to the initial therapy of plaque control, scaling and root planing. A high P.I. at a young age associated with low levels of plaque may well suggest Category E, as in Figure 10.1, but the clinician should be wary of hasty conclusions. In Fig. 10.1 the chart shows a high P.I. (4.3) in a young patient (28 years old). There is, however, good oral hygiene. These figures alone suggest Category E, but it is possible that the D.I. is low because the patient cleaned extra carefully just prior to the visit and usually has much worse plaque control. It is also possible that the high B.I. is due to active phases of the disease, and following scaling and root planing the periodontal pathology will respond to the therapy.

MONITORING CHART

Periodontal Control System

NAME __MRS S. SMITH__ AGE __28__

ASSESSMENT DATE: | 16 . 9 . 83 |

| | | 8 | 7 | ⑥ | 5 | 4 | 3 | 2 | 1 | ① | 2 | 3 | ④ | 5 | 6 | 7 | 8 |
| | | 8 | 7 | 6 | 5 | ④ | 3 | 2 | ① | 1 | 2 | 3 | 4 | 5 | ⑥ | 7 | 8 |

circle teeth used for DI and BI

CPITN

4	3	4
4	4	4

DEBRIS INDEX | 0 · 6 | BLEEDING INDEX | 0 · 9 |

INITIAL TREATMENT

Date	DI	BI
16 · 9 · 83	0 · 6	0 · 9
21 · 10 · 83	0 · 4	1 · 1

Date	DI	BI

Date	PI
21 · 10 · 83	4 · 3

SUGGESTED RECALL INTERVAL | |

LONG TERM CPITN ASSESSMENT
To be used as desired

Date _____ | | | |

Date _____ | | | |

Date _____ | | | |

Date _____ | | | |

Fig. 10.1   This is a typical chart of a susceptible patient who could well be Category E. The CPITN score considered against the patient's age is suspicious, and the relatively low D.I. (good oral hygiene) and high B.I. suggest an increased periodontal reaction to plaque. It is important to stress that a judgement about this patient cannot be made at the first visit. Many patients with this profile will respond to therapy. Only after a period of good plaque control without an improvement in disease levels can the patient be considered to be Category E.

After identification of the Category E patient a definite programme can be implemented as follows:

1. More frequent hygienist appointments (2-monthly).
2. In the absence of a suitable response to frequent scaling a 2 week course of metronidazole or tetracycline is prescribed. Metronidazole is usually the antibiotic of choice. If there is no improvement the clinician should consider the possibility of metronidazole-resistant organisms and the appropriate alternative is tetracycline.
3. In certain cases chlorhexidene gluconate mouthrinses for one or two weeks can be helpful. Some patients may find the Water-Pik a useful aid, whilst the deeply committed may be prepared to embark on subgingival irrigation using disposable syringes. One system combines an applicator for subgingival irrigation with the water-jet principle.
4. Very close monitoring of all indices is required following the pattern for Category D patients (as described in Chapter 11).

By using a carefully controlled and comprehensive pattern of treatment relying on frequent monitoring and therapy it is possible to maintain Category E patients for many years with minimal deterioration.

The Mechanics of a Recall System

As mentioned in Chapter 1 Kerr (7) found in his study in Aberdeen that most periodontal surgery failed in the absence of a suitable recall system. The provision of such a recall system can be time-consuming and awkward to implement.

Yet the caring practitioner must not only provide a suitable recall system but also ensure that his staff and hygienist carry it out. The system must provide a framework which allows the patient access to further periodontal care (usually in the form of scaling of selected areas, plaque control instruction and monitoring) within a suitable time-frame.

The interval that most studies seem to have settled on as being appropriate between recall visits is 3 months, but in some cases (especially the Category E patients) this can be too long. In our opinion there should be no definite time period but more a process of continuous review, using the 3-monthly recommendation as a basis and increasing or decreasing the interval as circumstances (and the indices) suggest.

The advantage of the monitoring forms (especially recording the D.I. and B.I.) becomes readily apparent. Using these 2 indices as a constant measure of the patient's oral hygiene and the inflammatory reaction to plaque gives either the dentist or hygienist the opportunity to advise the patient to increase or decrease the recall interval based on factual data rather than on a "feeling" about the clinical condition. These data can also be used to justify the clinical requirement for increasing the frequency of visits, either when seeking prior approval or when asking the patient for payment.

Summary

Certain patients fall into Category E and seem to be highly susceptible to a form of rapidly-progressing periodontal disease. It is possible to aid these patients in controlling their disease by frequent monitoring and scaling coupled with some form of antibacterial and chemical backup where appropriate.

Indications for this chemical backup can be provided by the indices which will show increasing deterioration (or failure to respond to therapy) despite good plaque control and traditional treatment in the form of scaling and non-surgical instrumentation.

References

1. Slots J. & Rosling B.G. (1983): Suppression of the periodontopathic microflora in localised juvenile periodontitis by systemic tetracycline. Journal of Clinical Periodontology 10 465-486.
2. Joyston-Bechal S., Smales F.C. & Duckworth R. (1984): Effect of metronidazole on chronic periodontal disease in subjects using a topically applied chlorhexidene gel. Journal of Clinical Periodontology 11 53-62.
3. Fine D.H., Letizia J. & Mandel I.D. (1985): The effect of rinsing with Listerine antiseptic on the properties of developing dental plaque. Journal of Clinical Periodontology 12 660-666.
4. Gordon J.M., Lamster I.B. & Seiger M.C. (1985): Efficacy of Listerine antiseptic in inhibiting the development of plaque and gingivitis. Journal of Clinical Periodontology 12 697-704.
5. Eakle W.S., Ford C. & Boyd R.L. (1986): Depth of penetration in periodontal pockets with oral irrigation. Journal of Clinical Periodontology 13 39-44.
6. Aziz-Gandour I.A. & Nerwman H.N. (1986): The effects of a simplified oral hygiene regime plus supragingival irrigation with chlorhexidene or metronidazole on chronic inflammatory periodontal disease. Journal of Clinical Periodontology 13 228-236.
7. Kerr N.W. (1981): Treatment of chronic periodontitis. British Dental Journal 150 222-224.

PART 4

SPECIAL CASES

This last section of the book deals with 2 special situations that can occur in general practice and which merit particular consideration. The first involves the patient who may benefit from periodontal surgery, and the second the patient who is not able to practise an adequate standard of plaque control.

The need for periodontal surgery can cause confusion within the mind of the general practitioner. Opinion as to whether or not surgery is indicated in typical cases with destructive disease seems to change with incredible frequency. The choice of the best procedure is also a matter of some discussion, as are the merits of non-surgical versus surgical treatment. The second subject, that of patient motivation, is one better suited to a separate book rather than simply a chapter. Most authorities constantly acclaim the importance of patient behaviour and dentist understanding, yet information about this vital topic is rare. We have restricted our discussion mainly to the role that monitoring can play in the orientation and motivation of the patient. This is because in the environment of a busy practice a method of using monitoring which can aid the motivation process is more relevant (though not more important) than a study of behaviour change, communication skills and the other topics which assist in our understanding of how to help patients motivate themselves.

Chapter 11

The Role of Surgery Now

Periodontal surgery has become a controversial topic in the last few years. Opinions range between the traditional view that scaling and oral hygiene acts as a pre-operative measure that prepares the mouth for the ultimate healing which will follow surgical intervention to an alternative view which embraces a concept of total non-surgical care.

The most appropriate course usually lies somewhere between the two opposing views, and for the general practitioner the main difficulty is knowing exactly what he should do for his patient in the light of the most recent knowledge. Should he continue to wait and assess before intervening surgically (which may mean a worsening of the situation for the patient) or should he intervene at once (and perhaps act hastily when continued scaling with monitoring would have been sufficient)?

As with many other aspects of periodontal care — monitoring by using the Periodontal Control System over a period of time will greatly assist in deciding whether to carry out surgery, and will also enable the longer term effects of surgical intervention to be established afterwards, a matter of equal importance.

Is Periodontal Surgery Ever Indicated?

The idea that periodontal surgery is a technique of doubtful value has arisen from a number of studies which seemed to suggest that if patients were reviewed several years after surgery there was little difference between areas of the mouth that had experienced surgery and areas where scaling alone had been the chosen treatment (1, 2, 3).

The concept of non-surgical care relies upon the fact that following careful root planing (and in some cases curettage of the pocket epithelium) the epithelium will attach to the root surface forming a "long epithelial attachment". Although this attachment appears to be less robust than the original fibrous attachment of the periodontal ligament when viewed in histological sections, clincally it is impossible to distinguish between the two in the presence of periodontal and gingival health. Thus pockets can be eliminated by a process of new attachment rather than by the removal of the soft tissue pocket wall (as in the gingivectomy procedure).

However in the studies mentioned above conclusions were being drawn

121

after averaging all the recordings of gingival inflammation and probing depths (in other words readings from shallow, medium and deep pockets were pooled). On closer examination of this kind of data it was found that if pockets were classified into shallow, medium and deep before analysis of the results, then the deep pockets were found to improve after surgery whilst the shallow pockets showed a deterioration (4). The averaging used in the earlier analyses had obscured the effect of depth and suggested that scaling and

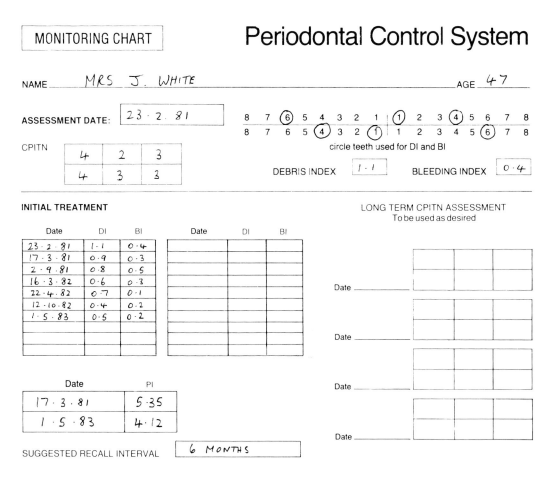

MONITORING CHART		Periodontal Control System			

NAME _MRS J. WHITE_ AGE _47_

ASSESSMENT DATE: _23 · 2 · 81_

8 7 (6) 5 4 3 2 1 | (1) 2 3 (4) 5 6 7 8
8 7 6 5 (4) 3 2 (1) | 1 2 3 4 5 (6) 7 8
circle teeth used for DI and BI

CPITN

4	2	3
4	3	3

DEBRIS INDEX _1·1_   BLEEDING INDEX _0·4_

INITIAL TREATMENT

Date	DI	BI
23·2·81	1·1	0·4
17·3·81	0·9	0·3
2·9·81	0·8	0·5
16·3·82	0·6	0·3
22·4·82	0·7	0·1
12·10·82	0·4	0·2
1·5·83	0·5	0·2

Date	DI	BI

LONG TERM CPITN ASSESSMENT
To be used as desired

Date _____

Date _____

Date	PI
17·3·81	5·35
1·5·83	4·12

Date _____

Date _____

SUGGESTED RECALL INTERVAL   _6 MONTHS_

Fig. 11.1.a   Monitoring Chart

This patient had an average oral hygiene score on her first visit (D.I. score of 1.1) which has improved to around 0.5 and been maintained over a 2 year period. Her P.I. score has reduced from 5.35 to 4.12 and is still high. Thus she is capable of maintaining good oral hygiene and has attended a regular recall system.

surgery produced equally beneficial effects on all pockets.

Thus the initial conclusion that surgical intervention was of limited value was erroneous. In reality deep pockets showed greater pocket reduction following surgery than after scaling alone. What the studies highlighted was the fact that medium pockets of 4-6mm, which previously would have automatically qualified for surgery, were now regarded as being suitably treated by careful scaling and root planing with reassessment.

When is Surgery Applicable?

Having decided that it is the deeper pockets which respond more favourably to a surgical approach, the next logical question is when should the procedure be undertaken. If it is done too soon, the surgery might fail, or even prove to be unnecessary; too late and further deterioration could occur.

With a careful system of monitoring this question is more easily answered. If the patient has good plaque control yet is still showing signs of disease in relation to the deep pockets then surgery should be planned. Such a case is illustrated in Figure 11.1.a, b and c.

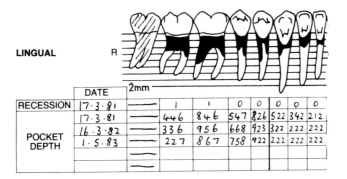

	DATE	2mm								
RECESSION	17·3·81	—	1		1		0	0	0	0	0
POCKET DEPTH	17·3·81	—	446	846	547	826	522	342	212
	16·3·82	—	336	956	668	923	322	222	222
	1·5·83	—	227	867	758	922	222	222	222

LINGUAL   R

Fig. 11.1.b   Probing Depth Chart

In the lower right quadrant the probing depths have not improved around the molars and premolars, in fact some have worsened.

Fig. 11.1.c (overleaf)   Distribution Chart

The plaque distribution shows an improvement in plaque removal around the teeth that have worsening pockets. This can be compared with the bleeding points which remain in the areas of deep pocketing.

Thus, this patient has continuing disease (bleeding on probing and pocket depths which have worsened) in the presence of good plaque control. She has also shown she will maintain regular visits (vital in aftercare following surgery). This is ideal for a successful outcome following surgery.

Periodontal Control System

NAME __MRS J. WHITE__   AGE __47__

PLAQUE DISTRIBUTION

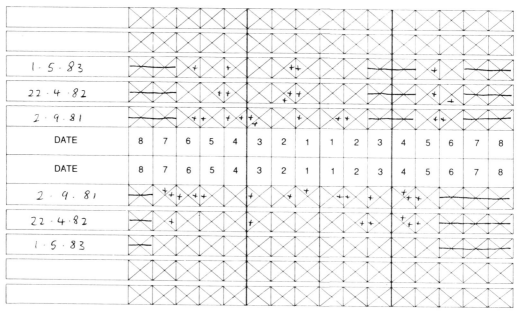

	8	7	6	5	4	3	2	1	1	2	3	4	5	6	7	8
1·5·83																
22·4·82																
2·9·81																
DATE	8	7	6	5	4	3	2	1	1	2	3	4	5	6	7	8
DATE	8	7	6	5	4	3	2	1	1	2	3	4	5	6	7	8
2·9·81																
22·4·82																
1·5·83																

BLEEDING POINTS DISTRIBUTION

	8	7	6	5	4	3	2	1	1	2	3	4	5	6	7	8
1·5·83																
16·3·82																
17·3·81																
DATE	8	7	6	5	4	3	2	1	1	2	3	4	5	6	7	8
DATE	8	7	6	5	4	3	2	1	1	2	3	4	5	6	7	8
17·3·81																
16·3·82																
1·5·83																

Study of the monitoring chart (Fig. 11.1.a) shows that the D.I. has reduced from 1.1 to around 0.5 and seems to be holding after a period of 2 years. The Probing Depths Chart (Fig. 11.1.b) shows several deep pockets around the teeth in the right quadrant which are staying at around 8-9 mm. Finally the Distribution Chart (Fig. 11.1.c) shows persistent bleeding on probing, and evidence of excellent plaque control in the lower right area.

These 3 features, good plaque control, deep pockets and persistent bleeding provide a definite indication for surgery. Thus in answer to the question of when to carry out surgery we can safely say that it is indicated when disease is continuing despite good levels of plaque control.

The Role of Aftercare

This topic has already been mentioned in Chapters 1 and 10 and is relevant here also. Surgery should not be considered unless the dentist can provide an adequate recall system to provide post-surgical care and monitoring and the patient is willing to partake in that recall programme. Studies by Axelsson & Lindhe and Kerr have demonstrated the importance of recall (5, 6).

Which Surgical Procedure is Best?

Once the need for surgery is established the choice of procedure confronts the practitioner. In the past the textbooks have provided details of a number of different techniques which tend to confuse rather than clarify.

In 1974 Kieser drew together many different lines of thought into a simple technique which he named the inverse bevel procedure (7). In this procedure a soft-tissue flap is raised to allow the operator to gain access to the roots underneath, sometimes with removal of a wedge of tissue around the teeth to resect some of the excess gingiva. After scaling and root planing the flap is replaced and sutured and allowed to heal. Minimal attempt is made to recontour bone as opinion now favours the view that the bone will remodel satisfactorily in the presence of meticulous post-surgical plaque control and regular visits for prophylaxis.

The other surgical technique which can be of value is the traditional gingivectomy procedure in areas of gingival overgrowth, where resection of excess tissue is all that is required.

Mucogingival Surgery

In the past mucogingival surgery has been used to re-establish the attached gingiva in the belief that a thick zone of attached gingiva helps to resist progression of the disease and aids in plaque control. Various studies have now challenged this belief, and current opinion favours the view that very little, or even no attached gingiva in the presence of good plaque control does not necessarily lead to deleterious effect.

Accordingly some of the earlier surgical techniques for restoring mucogingival anatomy (grafts, sliding flaps, etc.) are reserved for the rare case where aesthetics or a definite local deterioration indicates such treatment.

Summary

In the last few years there has been a definite shift in thinking away from the traditional concept of automatic surgical intervention to "remove" the diseased tissue and eliminate the pockets by resection towards a non-surgical approach which allows healing to occur by a new attachment of the tissues.

For the general practitioner faced with individual patients who require a decision on whether surgery is indicated or not, monitoring facilitates this decision by providing the necessary information in a clear and readable manner.

In the end, the final factor in any decision regarding surgery should be an assessment of the longterm prognosis, and with this in mind the provision of a post-surgical recall system is essential. The Periodontal Control System provides the vehicle to administer such a system.

References

1. Ramfjord P.R., Knowles, J.W., Nissle, R.R., Burgett, F.G. & Schick, R.A. (1975): Results following three modalities of periodontal therapy. Journal of Periodontology 46 522-526.

2. Knowles J., Burgett, F., Morrison, E., Nissle, R. & Ramfjord, S. (1980): Comparison of results following three modalities of periodontal therapy related to tooth type and initial pocket depth. Journal of Clinical Periodontology 7 32-47.

3. Badersten A., Nilvéus, R. & Egelberg, J. (1981): Effect of non-surgical therapy: 1. Moderately advanced periodontitis. Journal of Clinical Periodontology 8 57-72.

4. Pihistrom B.L., Ortiz-Campos, C. & Mettugh, R.B. (1981): A randomised 4-year study of periodontal therapy. Journal of Periodontology 52 227-242.

5. Kerr N.W. (1981): Treatment of chronic periodontitis. British Dental Journal 150 222-224.

6. Axelsson P. & Lindhe J., (1981): The significance of maintenance care in the treatment of periodontal disease. Journal of Clinical Periodontology 8 281-294.

7. Kieser J.B., (1974): An approach to periodontal pocket elimination. Brit. Journal of Oral Surgery 12 177-195.

8. Rosling B., Nyman, S., Lindhe, J. & Jern, B. (1976): The healing potential of the periodontal tissues following different techniques of periodontal surgery in plaque-free dentitions. Journal of Clinical Periodontology 3 233-250.

Chapter 12

What to do with the Patient Who Will Not Clean

One of the most difficult problems in the treatment of periodontal disease arises when the patient appears unable to practise plaque control to a level that is considered sufficient to control disease. Opinions have always varied on the best method of coping with this type of patient, varying from the one extreme of refusing to treat them at all to the other of ignoring the problem and providing treatment as if the plaque level was adequate.

In our view the skills of monitoring and motivation go hand in hand in helping to overcome the difficulty in this type of patient. These skills are powerful tools which help to create the desire for change within the patient that is so important.

Patient Motivation

Patient motivation is one of those subjects that is often talked about but rarely explained. The tendency in some books on dentistry, especially periodontology, is to make statements such as "... the patient must be sufficiently motivated ..." or "... once the patient has been motivated ..." without any positive help being given as to how this can be accomplished.

Clinicians recognise the importance of motivation but lack knowledge of how behavioural change occurs. This is hardly surprising, for the understanding of health behaviour requires extensive knowledge. Because this knowledge is formally taught under the headings of psychology, counselling, and interpersonal skills it is unlikely to be within the formal experience of most dentists and dental teachers.

Yet motivation is an extremely important subject for most dentists and their patients. Studies have shown that patients are more concerned about the interpersonal and social skills of their dentist than clinical and technical ability (1,2). Other studies have shown that inability to motivate is high on the list of anxieties experienced by dentists and similarly high on lists of the perceived needs of dental students and auxiliaries (3).

A Model for Behaviour Change

First we need to consider what motivation means. The dilemma is that patient motivation has different meanings for different people. This results in a number of alternative definitions in the textbooks and a few of these are given in Fig. 12.1.

129

1. Goal-directed energy that a patient expends.
2. Persuading people to do what you think is best for them.
3. The key to the achievement and maintenance of optimal oral hygiene.
4. The difference between a patient's goals and his perception of his level of achievement of those goals.

Fig. 12.1   Definitions of patient motivation.

The differences in emphasis create more difficulties in communication between dentist, hygienist, and patient. If the hygienist views motivation as achieving a behavioural change in the patient whilst the dentist assumes motivation to be the same as simply giving plaque control instruction there is likely to be a total breakdown in communication between the two with the result that the patient makes no progress.

Fig. 12.2 shows a model that can be used as a basic structure for achieving a change in the behaviour of a patient. By following the structure of the model we can see how motivation can be achieved and how the role of monitoring fits into the dental environment.

Finding the Patient's Goals

Before anyone is motivated to do anything at all they must perceive a suitable and attainable reward or reason. This reward may be in the nature of a negative reward or reinforcement (e.g. if you close the window the cold air will stop blowing down your neck) or more effectively it may be in the form of a positive one.

One of the first mistakes that dentists and hygienists can make is to assume that the patient's objectives are the same as their own. They then work on that assumption and use, say, the promise of healthy teeth for life as the incentive for carrying out the change in behaviour (flossing for example). If the patient's perception of healthy teeth for life is affected by experiences of their own and those of friends and family

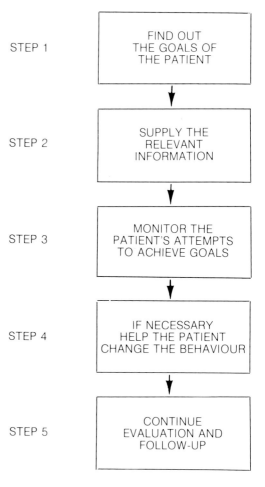

STEP 1 — FIND OUT THE GOALS OF THE PATIENT

STEP 2 — SUPPLY THE RELEVANT INFORMATION

STEP 3 — MONITOR THE PATIENT'S ATTEMPTS TO ACHIEVE GOALS

STEP 4 — IF NECESSARY HELP THE PATIENT CHANGE THE BEHAVIOUR

STEP 5 — CONTINUE EVALUATION AND FOLLOW-UP

Fig. 12.2   A model for behaviour change.

which suggest that it is most unlikely to be attained and will cause other problems (the cost of dental care, experiences of fillings that need replacing, for example), or if the patient just feels that teeth are a very low priority then motivation is unlikely to be accomplished.

Thus the first step in the motivation process is to discover what the patient's dental and oral goals are, and then if applicable to help them understand that those goals are possible, relevant and achievable.

Supplying the Relevant Information

Supplying information is not simply a matter of telling each patient everything they need to know because all of us find it difficult to absorb too much information at one time. Jargon (which is almost inevitable due to the familiarity that the dentist and hygienist acquire) causes an immediate breakdown in understanding, and many patients are afraid of wasting the dentist's time by asking questions.

A method of supplying information is to break down information into small, simple "packets" which are applicable to each individual patient. It is not necessary for the patient to understand the intimate details of the disease process to be told to use floss, but it is necessary for them to know why floss is important as opposed to just using a wood point.

In the process of giving information a tangible record of the patient's condition can be a valuable tool. Monitoring provides such a record as we will explain later in this chapter.

The Dentist/Patient Relationship

Besides the mechanics of behavioural change, we need to look at the relationship between patient and dentist, especially with regard to periodontal care. Traditionally the dentist/patient relationship has been one of teacher/pupil or parent/child. The dentist is regarded as the authority, giving help and advice to the patient who is regarded as the pupil. Because most dentists and hygienists are still taught their profession by authoritarian methods and in an authoritarian style they tend to regard their role of advisor in the same light. Their goal is to tell the patient what they (the advisor) knows is right. In simple terms, they need to tell the patient how to look after their teeth better and advise them how to do it. With conservative dentistry, in the management of dental pain, and in many other typical dental situations this approach is valid. The patient is definitely not the expert and help and advice followed by appropriate treatment will provide correct therapy. Once the tooth is extracted or filled the problem is dealt with and both patient and dentist can forget it. But in periodontal care we have a different situation.

Periodontal treatment requires more than the provision of correct therapy such as a filling or extraction. Because the patient plays a vital role in the longterm success, adjustment of the teacher/pupil relationship that exists in traditional dental relationships is required. For treatment to be successful the patient must take on the responsibility for those aspects of treatment which are carried out at home. Consequently the dentist/patient relationship needs to become one where both dentist and patient agree to work together in partnership towards the ultimate goal of periodontal health.

The Non-Authoritarian Approach

In the traditional authoritarian approach the patient comes for advice and the dentist or hygienist provides that advice. Both parties expect it and both feel happier afterwards. The patient is happy that his problem is solved (so he thinks) whilst the dentist is happy to have provided some help. Advice is quick to supply and costs the dentist little in time. The difficulty comes when the patient is expected to act on that advice, and this is often where the formula breaks down. Part of the reason may be that the advice given is applicable to the dentist's perception of the patient's needs rather than reality. The patient may not really want what the dentist thinks he needs, or may even pretend to want what the patient *thinks* the dentist would like.

The secret is for the dentist to discover what the patient *really* wants and then for the two of them to work together to find the best way of satisfying the *patient's* goals rather than the dentist's goals for the patient. This is formally known as the non-authoritarian approach.

There are disadvantages to this approach. It is more time-consuming and unfamiliar, both to dentist and patient. Trained by authoritarian methods the dentist feels uncomfortable when asking the patient to provide information about

his expectations and fears. The patient is also likely to feel uncomfortable at first as he is expecting to be "put right" which is a much easier solution than being asked that he has to start changing lifetime habits (such as diet and plaque control) to achieve what he wants. This unfamiliarity is likely to cause both parties to return to the authoritarian relationship so as to return to their comfort zones, with a resulting breakdown in the chances of success in health behaviour.

The Role of Monitoring

One of the main reasons why the non-authoritarian approach can break down is because of the lack of relevance perceived by the patient. Many people are puzzled when their dentist starts asking strange questions when he should really be "getting on with it".

However if a structure that appears familiar to the patient can be used to disguise the non-authoritarian approach success is more likely. The use of the monitoring forms provides just such a structure as they can be used to delve deeper into the patient's motives and goals without the patient being aware of the strategy.

We are not suggesting that the dentist and hygienist should continue with an authoritarian approach because both feel more comfortable using this type of approach. There is always more scope for better understanding and a deepening of the rapport so necessary for a good professional relationship. If the dentist takes time over several visits to discover more about the patient's feelings, expectations, desires and fears by careful open questioning, the relationship will be even better. What we are saying is that if either the dentist hygienist or patient finds this more open approach threatening, unfamiliar and uncomfortable then the monitoring charts can act as a useful vehicle and help the patient to discover what they really want and to communicate this to the dentist.

Monitoring the Patient's Attempts

Obviously this is where a monitoring chart becomes invaluable. To detect an improvement in plaque control using an agreed measure of plaque quantity is not only helpful, but is usually perceived by the patient as less threatening than the demonstration to the patient of areas of accumulated plaque within the patient's own mouth.

Because our society is used to considering figures on paper as measures of self-assessment the chart is more acceptable as a messenger of bad news rather than the more colourful descriptions given by the dentist to the patient. Attempts to identify areas that the patient is "missing" by using plaque disclosing techniques and direct vision can create tensions within the patient which will act as barriers to further communication. Often the apparently innocent process of showing patients the areas in the mouth they are failing to clean is perceived by the patient as being "told off" no matter how gently it is done.

Fig. 12.3 shows a simple plaque score (the meaning of the figures is irrelevant to the exercise) which indicates to both

DEBRIS INDEX

Date

12.3.81	1.2
29.3.81	0.9
16.9.81	0.8
23.10.81	0.6
8.6.82	0.8
9.12.82	0.5
20.7.83	0.4

Fig. 12.3   The Debris Index

the operator and patient that plaque control is improving.

Even more productive is the situation which occurs if the figures show a deterioration. As soon as the concerned patients sees the figures worsen they will be prompted to enquire as to how matters can be improved, creating an ideal environment for further plaque control instruction or other advice. This helpful situation is not created so readily in the classic confrontation between dentist (or hygienist) and patient, when the one has to tell the other it is their opinion that they are not cleaning as well as they should. This can often set up resistant barriers within the patient — no matter how calm they appear on the surface.

Continuing Evaluation and Follow-Up

One of the most difficult tasks faced by the dentist carrying out periodontal therapy is to remember the condition of the gingiva and the level of plaque control over a period of years. However, for

133

motivation to continue it is essential that this very information be provided to the patient for long-term feedback effects to occur.

With the passage of time the patient's newly-acquired skills in oral hygiene will become established and there will be less necessity for strict monitoring. The annual reminders and checking can continue to serve as useful prompts throughout the patient's life.

EXAMPLE

Mr. J. Black, aged 43

Mr. J. Black attended for an examination. The CPITN chart showed the following:

4	2	3
2	2	2

On the strength of this information Mr. Black was placed into Category D. The D.I. and B.I. were measured, resulting in a preliminary Monitoring Chart as in Fig. 12.4

The information in Fig. 12.4 suggested that Mr. Black's plaque control is average and will need improving. There is inflammation present (the B.I. score of 0.8) and the CPITN score shows pocketing in both upper posterior sextants. After 2 more visits which involved mainly plaque control instruction and scaling the chart looked like Fig. 12.5.

At the completion of treatment the D.I. and B.I. have both reduced and the patient is advised to continue cleaning.

134

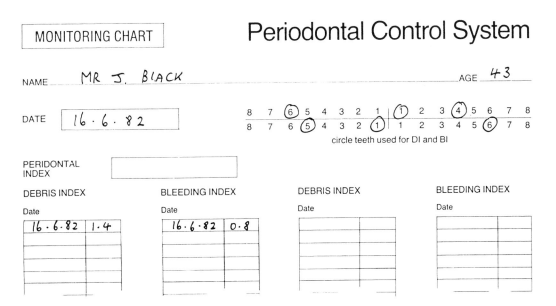

Fig. 12.4 D.I. and B.I. at 1st visit.

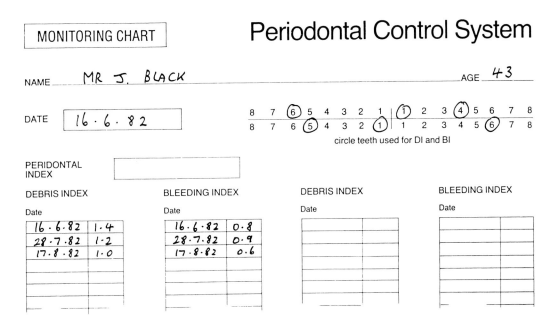

Fig. 12.5 D.I. and B.I. after two months.

EXAMPLE

6 Months Later

The CPITN was taken again and showed little change apart from the lack of

4	1	3
2	2	2

calculus in one sextant. The most disappointing finding was that both the D.I. and the B.I. were worse than on the first visit (see Fig. 12.6).

At this stage the patient's inability to practise adequate plaque control could be demonstrated using the figures, and this can lead to a discussion on what the patient really wants (the non-authoritarian approach). From this discussion the dentist begins to understand how best to help Mr. Black, and the patient begins to perceive that treatment is more than simple advice and scaling (a view often held by patients).

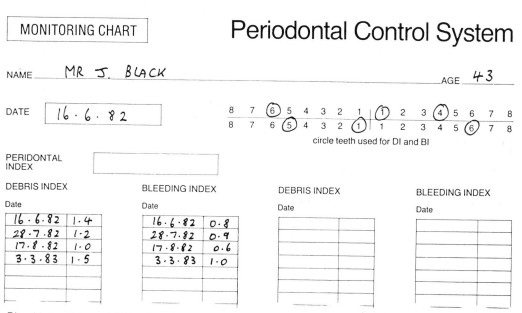

Fig. 12.6   D.I. and B.I. relapsing after 9 months.

| MONITORING CHART | | Periodontal Control System |

NAME   MR J. BLACK   AGE   43

DATE   16 . 6 . 82

8 7 ⑥ 5 4 3 2 1 | ① 2 3 ④ 5 6 7 8
8 7 6 ⑤ 4 3 2 ① | 1 2 3 4 5 ⑥ 7 8
circle teeth used for DI and BI

PERIDONTAL INDEX

DEBRIS INDEX

Date	
16 . 6 . 82	1 . 4
28 . 7 . 82	1 . 2
17 . 8 . 82	1 . 0
3 . 3 . 83	1 . 5

BLEEDING INDEX

Date	
16 . 6 . 82	0 . 8
28 . 7 . 82	0 . 9
17 . 8 . 82	0 . 6
3 . 3 . 83	1 . 0

DEBRIS INDEX

Date

BLEEDING INDEX

Date

The Role of Scaling

Despite the best efforts of the dentist to communicate the need for good oral hygiene some patients will never improve. In certain rather rare circumstances this may not matter (for example the older patient with large amounts of plaque, no periodontal pocketing and little inflammation) and in our opinion the presence of plaque alone in the absence of disease is not a matter of concern. Such patients require monitoring to ensure that damage does not occur if the cyclic nature of the disease suddenly emerges, but if disease is absent then immediate attempts to help the patient motivate himself are unnecessary.

This does not excuse the dentist from taking any action whatsoever, and such patients can benefit from scaling and plaque instruction by having a "fresher" and cleaner mouth. The indices will ensure that both the patient and the dentist are fully aware of what is happening and can take effective action should a change occur.

The difficulty arises when the patient is failing to carry out adequate plaque control and there is evidence of active disease (as in the case of Mr. Black outlined above). If there is little or no response after a period of time and the patient continues to fail in his plaque control efforts then some dentists would advocate withdrawal from the situation. The attitude tends to be one of "If the patient can't be bothered then why should I?"

This is understandable from 2 points of view. Firstly the dentist may well have other patients who are all practising excellent plaque control and thus more deserving of his or her attention, and if time is at a premium then these patients must take preference. Secondly, and of more importance if it is true, if treatment of any sort *in the absence of good plaque control* proves to be ineffectual then until the patient does motivate himself any further action on the part of the dentist (other than of an emergency nature) would be a waste of time.

The first argument, that other patients should take precedence, is a matter of personal opinion which we feel unable to comment upon. However the second point is crucial in the argument and is not open to debate as evidence for the efficacy of scaling alone in the absence of plaque control does exist.

Lovdal et al showed that scaling helped patients with poor plaque control in their early work on the effects of scaling and supervised plaque control (4) and other workers have also shown that relatively speaking the role of scaling is much more important than the role of home-care (5). However in one study some patients were scaled *in the absence of any plaque control instruction at all* and were compared with patients who received plaque control instruction plus scaling (6). Although the patients receiving both showed greater disease reduction, scaling alone had a significant effect. Thus we feel justified in stressing that even in the absence of *any* patient cooperation in plaque control, continued scaling of the mouth will have beneficial effects and should always be provided if the patient is willing.

137

Summary

We have discussed, albeit briefly, some of the basic steps required in establishing a behaviour change in a patient, often referred to as patient motivation.

The problem of the patient who will not cooperate in taking the responsibility of adequate homecare can seem insurmountable to the busy practitioner and hygienist. Amongst the many factors leading to non-cooperation is the difficulty of finding out just what the patient wants. If this is not done the dentist simply gives advice which he or she suspects is related to the patient's wishes.

Monitoring is helpful in demonstrating in a non-threatening fashion that the patient needs assistance if disease is not responding, and also provides a "trigger" which enables the dentist to enquire further into the patient's true wishes. The charts also provide tangible goals which dentist and patient can aim for (such as a D.I. score of 0.5).

Even if this approach fails and the patient still refuses to change his plaque control pattern significantly enough to restore health, there is sufficient evidence to show that, providing the patient is prepared to attend, a regular programme of scaling will be of definite benefit. This may require a change in attitude of the dentist and hygienist who have often been taught that such a patient is not worth bothering about.

References

1. Kriesberg L. & Treiman, B.R. (1962). Dentists and the practice of dentistry as viewed by the public. Journal of American Dental Association 64 806-821.
2. Hellman V., (1972). 8 Reasons why your patients won't be back. Dental Economics 62. 22-26.
3. Ingersoll T.G., Ingersoll B.D., Seime R.J. & McCutcheon W.R. (1978). A survey of patients and auxiliary problems as they relate to behavioural dentistry curricula. Journal of Dental Education 42 260-263.
4. Lovdal A., Arnö, A., Shei, O. & Waerhaug, J. (1961): Combined effect of sub-gingival scaling and controlled plaque control on the incidence of gingivitis. Acta Odontologica Scandinavica 19 537-553.
5. Cercek J.F., Kiger R.D., Garrett S. & Egelberg J. (1983): Relative effects of plaque control and instrumentation on the clinical parameters of human periodontal disease. Journal of Clinical Periodontology 10 46-56.
6. Chawla T.N., Nanda R.S. & Kapoor K.K. (1975): Dental prophylaxis procedures in control of periodontal disease in Lucknow (rural) India. Journal of Periodontology 46 498-503.

Afterword

We have shown a system of monitoring patients in general practice which we believe to be of immense practical help to the dentist and hygienist wishing to provide a system of continuing care within the framework of a general practice.

This system has been named the Periodontal Control System because it gives the operator much more control over the diagnosis, treatment and prognosis of periodontal disease. Using the 4 basic charts provided within the Periodontal Control System it is possible to monitor patients for many years and remain confident that the disease is truly under control. The discipline of taking a form of index on a regular basis also provides the framework for continued motivation for the patient.

Although the aetiology, prevalence and severity of periodontal disease is still uncertain there is no doubt amongst all authorities that provision of plaque control and a change in the behaviour of patients is the most effective method of treatment. The concept of an acceptable level of plaque being tolerated by the patient to enable them to keep the disease under control is also an attractive one, as is the identification of both patients who are "high risk" and areas of disease within each dentition. A system such as the Periodontal Control System also provides a suitable method for all these points.

Finally the difficulty of provision of such a system within the "fee for item of service" structure must also be considered. Once again, whilst not ideal, the Periodontal Control System solves this by enabling justification of the fee (either to the patient or the ultimate provider of the payment, be it Insurance Company or State).

We are not advocating that the Periodontal Control System is the perfect answer to all periodontal care. What we are sure of is that this system has been proved to be effective in many dental practices in the United Kingdom already, and besides being of practical value also answers many of the theoretical and academic recommendations for the provision of periodontal care today.

Index